RELATIONAL REFLEXOLOGY

THE BLOG POSTS

NICHOLA GREGORY

Relational Reflexology The Blog Posts © 2014 Nichola Gregory

All Rights Reserved. No part of this publication may be reproduced, stored in a retrieval system, or transmitted, in any form or in any means, by electronic, mechanical, photocopying, recording or otherwise, without prior written permission.

Disclaimer:

The information contained in this book is not intended to serve as a replacement for professional medical advice. Any use of the information in this book is done so at the reader's discretion. The author and publisher specifically deny any and all liability arising directly or indirectly from the use or application of any information contained in this book. A health care professional should always be consulted regarding any specific situation.

First Printing, 2014

ISBN-13: 978-1500530914

ISBN-10: 1500530913

RELATIONAL REFLEXOLOGY

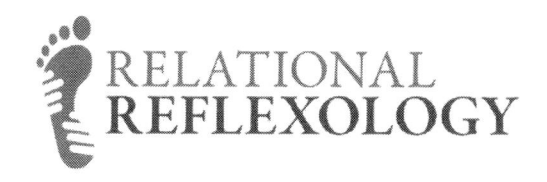

For Cameron

With Love

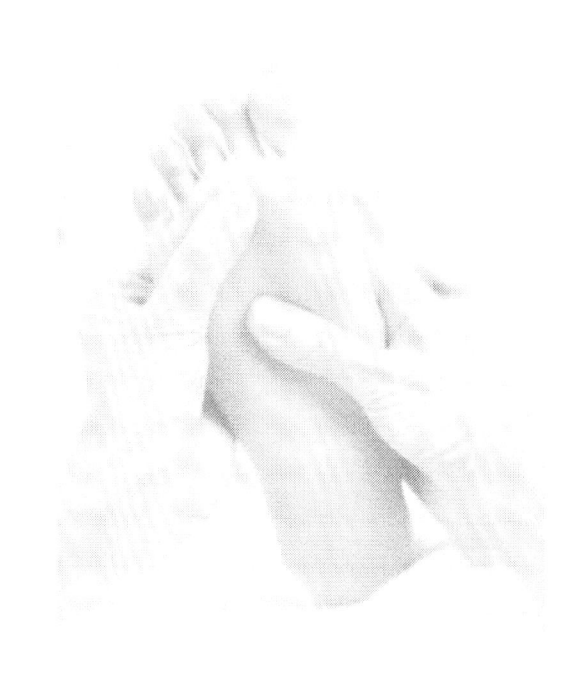

Contents

INTRODUCTION 1

THE SEPARATION OF MIND AND BODY IN HEALTH
A HISTORICAL PERSPECTIVE 11

REFLEXOLOGY? THAT'S ALL ABOUT THE FEET, RIGHT? 21

REFLEXOLOGY FLAVOURS 25

REFLEXOLOGY – A THERAPEUTIC ART FORM, NOT A PROCEDURE 27

VERBAL COMMUNICATION AND CLIENT EMOTIONAL DISCLOSURE
PRACTITIONER SURVEY FINDINGS 31

A PLACE FOR LOVE IN REFLEXOLOGY? 45

THE MULTI-DIMENSIONAL IMPACT
OF INTERPERSONAL TOUCH IN REFLEXOLOGY 51

WIRED FOR COMPASSION – THE HUMAN BRAIN
AND THE SUPPORTIVE REFLEXOLOGY PACKAGE 67

THE BRAIN, ELECTRICAL IMPULSES,
CHEMICAL COMMUNICATIONS AND REFLEXOLOGY 79

TO TREAT OR NOT TO TREAT, THAT IS THE QUESTION
FEAR AND CONTRAINDICATION IN REFLEXOLOGY 111

PHILOSOPHY AND WELL-BEING IN REFLEXOLOGY 121

MEETING STRESS, ANXIETY, PANIC AND DEPRESSION IN REFLEXOLOGY ... 127

THE THERAPEUTIC RELATIONSHIP IN REFLEXOLOGY 133

PRACTITIONER SELF DEVELOPMENT	139
WINNIE THE POOH PSYCHOLOGY - A REFLECTIVE PRACTITIONER EXERCISE	143
POWER AND RESPONSIBILITY IN THE REFLEXOLOGY RELATIONSHIP	153
THE FELT SENSE, INTERPRETATION AND MINDFULNESS IN REFLEXOLOGY	161
EXTERNALISING IN REFLEXOLOGY - GIVING EMOTIONS SHAPES AND COLOURS	173
DEVELOPING A THERAPEUTIC VOCABULARY IN REFLEXOLOGY	177
REFLEXOLOGY AND THE WHOLE PERSON - INTERSTITIAL CYSTITIS	187
REFLEXOLOGY AND THE WHOLE PERSON - CHRONIC HEADACHE AND MIGRAINE	197
REFLEXOLOGY AND THE WHOLE PERSON - VERTIGO, TINNITUS, AND LABYRINTHITIS	205
CLINICAL INFORMATION RELATING TO SUB-FERTILITY	217
THE EMOTIONAL IMPACT OF SUB-FERTILITY	233
REFLEXOLOGY AND THE WHOLE PERSON - SUB-FERTILITY	237
TCM PHILOSOPHY AND REFLEXOLOGY	255
AN OPEN LETTER TO THE BEAUTY AND SPA WORLD	265
HOPE AND CLOSING REFLECTIONS	269
REFERENCES	275
USEFUL LINKS	285

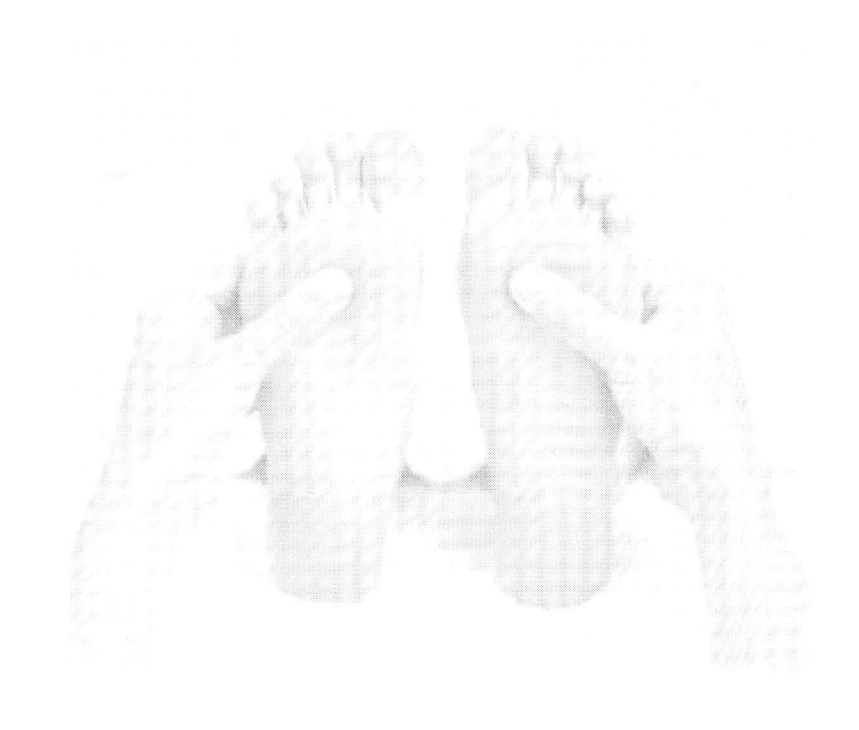

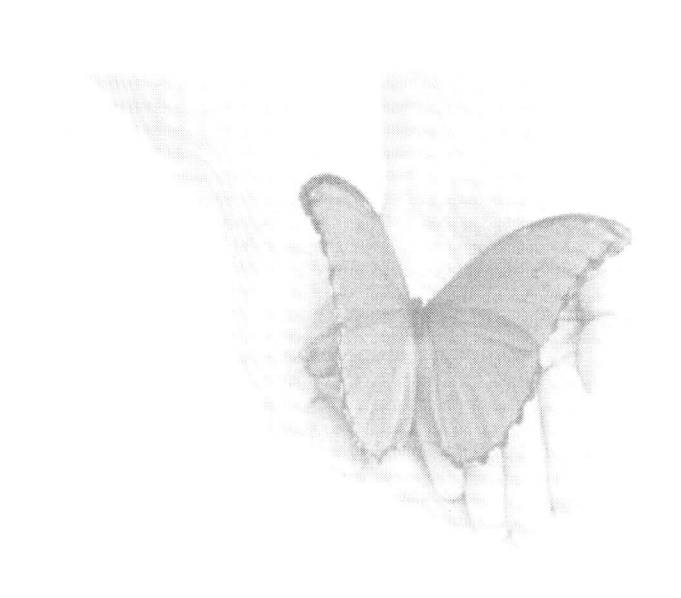

Introduction

"The true lover of knowledge naturally strives for truth, and is not content with common opinion, but soars with undimmed and unwearied passion till he grasps the essential nature of truth."

- Plato

Have you ever attempted to construct a jigsaw puzzle without the box lid as a reference guide? Perhaps a fairly slow, frustrating, confusing endeavour? The supportive reflexology package might be likened to the holistic version of a 500 piece jigsaw puzzle - without a box lid!

Scientific investigations examine one piece of the jigsaw at a time, so as to formulate a more detailed understanding of the phenomenon under investigation. However, most researchers tend also to work within a framework of **hypotheses** – a hypothesis is a bit like the researchers jigsaw puzzle box lid, only in black and white. It's a possibility, an idea, an impression.

Hypotheses - Noun

A supposition, or proposed explanation, made on the basis of limited evidence as a starting point for further investigation.

Hypotheses - Philosophy

A proposition made as a basis for reasoning, without any assumption of its truth.

Some of the information presented in this book represents my own basic personal **hypotheses** for why many clients can report positive therapeutic outcomes to reflexology treatment, across multi-dimensional realms (mind and body). The information represents my own *black and white* interpretation of the reflexology puzzle box lid.

The 500 piece jigsaw can often appear far more detailed on completion than might have ever been imagined initially. The completed puzzle displays in deep, rich, and vibrant colour. It will take on a more multi-dimensional, complex, and detailed appearance. In essence the picture will come to life!

The Reflexology Puzzle

In order to better understand the detail within any phenomenon, it is important to first formulate a basic description of how that phenomenon appears.

The reflexology puzzle box lid clearly shows a picture of two people sitting closely together, hands and feet are clearly visible in the picture, one person is undoubtedly touching the other, and there seems to be a verbal exchange occurring. Indeed it's a picture of many parts.

If we could zoom into that picture, and perhaps even into the feet themselves we might certainly become aware of *other* complex jigsaw puzzles:

- **Communications occurring between the feet and the brain.**

- **Communications occurring between the toucher and the touched.**

If we could understand what was being exchanged within the verbal interactions of the two people yet another complex jigsaw would emerge:

- **One person's reactions to experiencing a listening, supportive ear.**

There are many aspects involved in a supportive reflexology encounter.

Politics and Reflexology

In the UK, as a growing CAM industry, reflexology has taken some great leaps forward in terms of structuring professional standards. Over a number of years the reflexology federal working group formulated and agreed upon the core curriculum for reflexology, and defined our National Occupational Standards.

That work (and work from other modalities) led to the eventual forming of the Complementary and Natural Healthcare Council (CNHC) set up with government funding in 2008 to act as the UK voluntary regulator for complementary healthcare practitioners.

As a result of this enormous combined effort, today in the UK, the minimum level of reflexology training recognised by the established professional reflexology associations now stands at Level 3, with entry level training in some cases up to Level 5. Unfortunately however, any phenomenon identified as a potentially viable commodity fairly soon feels the firm hand of definition and control. Reflexology is now undoubtedly in that place.

Recent advertising restrictions (affecting the UK), have resulted in practitioners being forced to sanitise wording within their reflexology practice adverts. Nothing is real anymore - *apparently* - until vigorously and quantifiably studied! Additionally, the advertising regulators have recommended before making any future modality 'claims' reflexology should to meet some fairly hefty criteria related to producing a large and *'acceptable'* body of clinical, quantifiable, type evidence - or double blind trials.

I have to admit to feeling more than a little frustrated that the voice of the *'official line'* in reflexology seems to have been allocated to a form of research closely associated with the medical model. The medical model, whilst entirely capable of identifying useful clinical applications for the modality, and undoubtedly helpful in terms of identifying the physiological impact of reflexology, is simply not constructed to fully comprehend, or research, the many complexities associated with a supportive reflexology exchange

Reflexology Research

Any study examining a certain aspect of reflexology represents a single piece of a much larger jigsaw puzzle. Encouragingly, professional reflexology practitioners are increasingly engaging in impressive and entirely useful clinical research studies. Here in the UK, for instance, we are immensely proud of resent research undertaken by Dr. Carol Samuel, who published a study in 2013 examining the impact of reflexology on acute pain responses, and also Sally Kay, who studied reflexology's impact on lymphatic drainage. Both studies demonstrated impressive results. Well constructed studies such as these certainly help to demonstrate clinical applications for reflexology (i.e. pain management/lymphatic drainage), and will undoubtedly only positively influence any application to source addition funding for research in a similar area. These studies additionally assist in highlighting, and giving context to, a single piece of the complex reflexology puzzle.

Understanding Research Methodologies

Quantitative (or quantifiable) research is involved with gathering data which is absolute, such as numerical data, so it can be counted and modelled statistically. Quantitative tests are designed to remove as much bias as possible, are often randomised, and the information collated would be expected to remain consistent should the test be carried out repeatedly. This type of research is closely aligned with the *classical scientific paradigm*.

Qualitative research, on the other hand, is a much more *subjective* form of research enquiry. Often the data collected from a qualitative study will yield little concrete data in the form of numbers, but instead might focus on experience, stories, feelings and emotions. The researcher accepts bias as a natural part of a qualitative enquiry, accepting it can form a more complete picture. Studies are often presented as case study, as they allow for a richer, more detailed account of the subject. Certainly, there exists great debate regarding the *validity* of qualitative studies within the field of social sciences, with some researchers suggesting more rigorous studies should be adopted, so that results can more generalised and therefore gain acknowledgment from the wider clinical community. Equally, there are those who wholeheartedly believe individual human experience simply cannot be quantified.

The Problem with Blinding

"Not everything that can be counted counts and not everything that counts can be counted. - William Bruce Cameron

One important tenet related to randomised controlled trials (*double blind trials*) relates to attempting to eliminate/reduce *bias*. In order to promote objectivity participants ideally should remain uninfluenced by prior expectation. One way researchers try to avoid bias manifesting in research trials is to refrain from revealing group allocation to participants (i.e. real pill group/sugar pill group). Researchers call this process of eliminating bias **blinding**.

In a **double blind** trial the main aim is to keep *everyone* involved participant/researcher/data collection support) from knowing a participants allocation group. This is certainly a relatively simple stance to achieve in a trial examining, for instance, medication. Blinding in a reflexology study might be used help to narrow focus on the mechanics of action, or to attempt to identify the benefit of utilising one particular reflex over another (sham reflex, or sham reflex points). Clearly, one of the main limitations involved in this type of study relates to the manner in which the reflexology treatment/session might compare to the form of reflexology occurring within most therapy rooms. Can one ever possibly hope to separate the influence of the individual practitioner, or the dynamics of an interpersonal interaction, from the underlying mechanics of reflexology? Can the intention contained within the touch of a caring, supportive reflexologist simply be deposited at the research room door, or eliminated entirely from the equation? Research stemming from the fields of social psychology and neuroscience would seem to suggest not. Rather, touch scientists inform us human beings are capable of communicating up to eight different emotions through their use of touch, and that the impact of touch is directly related to the individual's social evaluation of the person providing it. Surely this connection between two people is as much related to the art of reflexology as the relationship between the hands and feet, or the feet and brain? In that case we might be wise to also begin to consider the intimate relational aspect of many reflexology sessions, and the potential impact of encountering a supportive educational relationship; a safe place in which to learn to relax and just 'be'.

Measuring the Unique Human Individual

"The things that make me different are the things that make me." - A.A. Milne

In summary, it would seem the *mechanics* of reflexology, and the impact of the *reflexology package* can be defined quite separately. The first (mechanics) represents an integral part of a much larger whole. Therefore, perhaps the ideal reflexology research structure might be mixed methodology; a study both open enough to appreciate the whole and unique (**qualitative**), whilst remaining detailed enough to demonstrate more solid clinical type measurements (**quantitative**).

Research in the Private Sector

Unfortunately, a gathering of good quality information relating to how reflexology is experienced more generally by the public, or indeed practiced within the private sector, does not currently exist. Many reflexology studies have previously focused, for instance, on investigations utilising *sham* reflexology points. Information presented in the interpersonal touch article demonstrates why studies such as these are unsuitable; the therapeutic impact of touch alone is just too enormous. Some studies have looked at outcomes with specific client groups, unfortunately often without having first theoretically factored in the many complexities of the reflexology exchange; results therefore tend to be inconclusive. Additionally, in order for research to be published, and therefore acknowledged, it must meet a certain standard of criteria. Many previous reflexology studies have simply not been constructed appropriately.

Given the vast majority of reflexology is occurring within the private sector it would seem sensible for the industry to begin to establish sound, acceptable research methodologies, and to begin to build our own body of good quality research, rather than wait to rely upon what *might* emerge from the clinical world. We must come to accept clinically based reflexology research is motivated entirely by health sector requirements, and very real funding limitations, and certainly not by an altruistic desire to help define reflexology. The health sector pot of research money is often allocated to important medical type research long before complementary therapies are considered. Perhaps we have been a little naive in believing if we waited for long enough the clinical world would finally acknowledge the worth of reflexology, and help us out! The clinical world has its own agenda, and whilst reflexology can certainly play some part within that agenda, we would be foolish to believe from that place reflexology will eventually come to be recognised for all its therapeutic worth.

Moving Forward

Reflexology is complex, powerful, and entirely underestimated, by almost everyone, except practitioners, and our clients. Perhaps now is time to collectively begin to change that reality and take responsibility for the future reputation and life force of the wonderful *art* of reflexology. The key to building a good and valid body of research evidence is to initially begin to collate a sound body of detailed case study work. Case study work can then provide context with which to approach, for instance, associated charity and support groups, to request funding for more detailed studies. For the moment reflexology based research studies should try to focus on identifying useful 'gaps' in the market. That is to identify areas in which it is possible to really demonstrate the positive impact of reflexology and to provide a useful therapeutic intervention to those clients benefiting from funding.

The concept of engaging in reflexology research, or even attempting to make sense of scientific research papers or academic information, can feel overwhelming for many reflexology practitioners. My hope is some of the information in the blog articles will start to familiarise the reader with a few of the more common terms utilised within research and academia, and that through this familiarisation process an increasing number of practitioners will feel more confident about the possibility of engaging in well constructed research studies. To support us in this task we are fortunate in the UK to have among us individuals such as Tracey Smith - Reflexology and Research Manager at the Association of Reflexologists, and, Judith Whatley - Senior Lecturer at Cardiff Metropolitan University. Tracey's extensive knowledge base and previous career as a scientist places her in the perfect position to straddle two very different worlds. Judith's career centres round understanding reflexology research, and supporting reflexology researchers. These are the people best placed to guide practitioners in private practice in terms of reflexology research. Research does not have to be complicated; it simply needs to be well constructed. Tracey and Judith can certainly assist practitioners in this area.

Summary

Whilst the feet, hands, and ears are centrally placed in reflexology there are *other* important elements within our therapeutic interactions also worth acknowledgment - *other pieces of the jigsaw*. The intention therefore in compiling the articles contained within this book is to:

1. **Offer a detailed phenomenological account of the manner in which reflexology might be more generally practiced with the private sector.**

2. **Acknowledge the importance of the practitioner's role within the supportive reflexology package and highlight the relational aspect of reflexology**

3. **Draw attention to the associated importance of practitioner self development.**

4. **Highlight the necessity to develop more holistic and kaleidoscopic research studies capable of fully appreciating the complex multi-dimensional impact of the reflexology package.**

Housekeeping

I am aware there may be some readers of the blog (and this book) curious to understand why I tend not to refer to specific reflex areas in the feet? I try to write for qualified reflexologists, and so I am aware most readers are already quite proficient in carrying out the physical application of reflexology - I have no desire to teach the reader to suck eggs! Additionally, my interest lies more in championing the multi-dimensional impact of the reflexology package. I am therefore happy to leave discussions concerning subjects such as the specific location of reflex points, or how best to work the points, to those practitioners more captured by these particular aspects of reflexology.

It is a rare occurrence for a client to attend my practice these days without an accompanying diagnosed condition. Most of the reflexology work I engage in falls into three distinct categories: chronic anxiety, sub-fertility, and migraine. Therefore, the tone of my writing is reflective of the form of reflexology I personally tend to practice, and certainly not wholly representative of *every* reflexology experience.

The original blog posts presented within the book emerged organically across a seven month period. I have restructured the sequence in which they appear here, as well as including additional material, so as to provide the reader with a more naturally flowing text.

And finally, I genuinely hope you find something useful here to add to your own reflexology tool box.

.

Relational Reflexology

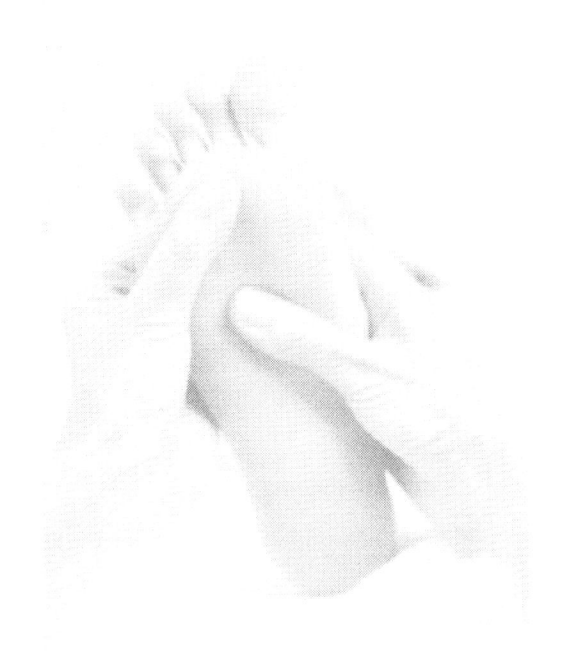

The Separation of Mind and Body in Health
A Historical Perspective

"Declare the past, diagnose the present, foretell the future."

- Hippocrates

The concept of ancient health and medicine can sometimes appear mysterious and difficult to comprehend to modern day man, particularly when attempts are made to measure the Ancient's knowledge by the intellectual, scientific models and standards of today. The formation and growth of modern medicine can be traced back across thousands of years; its development encouraged by more settled human societies, religion, philosophy, education, trade, and of course, the ever enquiring human mind. Latterly, with so many astonishing advances occurring within science and modern medicine it might be perhaps easy to imagine that human beings could only have gained with regards to their health. Whilst scientific achievements are undoubtedly of tremendous value to the entire human race, it could also be argued along its developmental journey both science and modern medicine became, *for a time*, somewhat blinded to fully appreciating the complex human condition, and the innate and subtle interactions between mind and body.

Pre-History

Pre-literate man left us no written record of his knowledge of the body, health or medicines, although anthropologists have been able to make some associations with modern-day cultures such as the Australian Aborigines, who until the late eighteenth century remained entirely isolated from the outside world, yet were discovered to be relatively healthy (Graham, 1999). It is believed many pre-historic tribes believed in animism; a concept stating that individual lives and the functions of the human body were influenced by, and at the mercy of, unpredictable spirits. Belief systems such as these placed the Shaman, or witch doctor, at the centre of tribal nomadic life. The Shaman was viewed as a master of divination, healing, foresight and interpretation.

The Shaman could communicate with the spirit world. He possessed mastery over fire and rain, and he could journey in varying altered states of consciousness for the purpose of diagnosis, prophecy or insight. Whereas in the modern sense illness and disease might be viewed as external agents affecting the body, to these ancient pre-historic and shamanic cultures illness was essentially considered a spiritual matter; one principally believed to stem from a loss of individual personal power, with disease considered as originating and gaining meaning from the spiritual.

Ancient Egypt

The emergence of the great human civilisations and the growing exploration of the wider world meant a more structured concept of healing soon began to emerge. The ancient Egyptians were perhaps the first to embrace and formalise the concept of medicine and healing. Increased stability stemming from more settled farming economies encouraged the development of formalised governments, laws and social norms, as well as sparking the emergence of structured religious practices and the invention of writing and calculation. The significant development of writing meant rather than relying on verbal tradition alone for passing on knowledge, ideas could be now be recorded and developed for further study and education. Medicine however was still deeply rooted in the magical and the divine and the healer priests of the time were highly regarded as the holders and keepers of ancient sacred wisdom.

The Egyptians viewed their very existence as being intrinsically connected to the workings of the universe, and often directly to the working of their Gods. To the ancient Egyptians the universe existed in perfect energetic harmony, with man considered as a perfect microcosm and representation of that harmony.

As well as colour and rhythm existing as important healing tools, higher status priests were also said to be able to tap into and direct natural universal energies and they were particularly interested in energies emanating from the sun (or Ra). Healer priests sought to direct energy from the sun directly to their patient, and so practiced the passing of hands over the body, in an attempt to invoke changes in the subtle etheric energy (or spiritual body); believing the energy would be absorbed into the more vital, physical elements of the individual, thus inducing a state of both spiritual and physical healing.

The temple priests also made use of herbs and spices brought back by traders from all over the known world, and the practice of mummification encouraged a deeper understanding of the body and its internal organs.

The Egyptian concept of channel theory emerged after temple priests observed damage occurring in farmer's fields when irrigation channels became blocked. The principle was also utilised as a source of understanding disease within the human body. The development of this more formalised theory of human health began to signify Egyptian Gods were no longer being perceived as entirely responsible for human illness, and the healer priests of the time began to strive towards finding more physical interventions to restore the health of mind, body (and spirit).

Ancient Greece

The ancient Greek civilisations began to emerge just as the Egyptian age began to fade. Above all it might be said the Greeks liked to think. They placed importance on the concept of rational and logical thinking, striving always to understand why things happen, and so under the Ancient Greeks, the art of philosophy prospered. The concepts of harmony, right balance and measure were of central importance to Greek philosophers, and their main aim until the sixth century BC was understanding *physis;* the attempt to perceive the essential and true nature of all things.

According to Greek myth, Asclepius, son of the god Apollo and the nymph Coronis, was born from the dead body of his mother. Asclepius was raised by Chiron, a centaur, who was considered a master of medical practice and herbal medicine. Soon Asclepius surpassed his master's knowledge and became known as the Greek God of medicine. Over 200 temples to Asclepius's were constructed, representing the first known hospitals. Patients were permitted to rest and to sleep in the temples, where they believed through dreams and insight they might perceive the presence of the Asclepius, who would provide therapeutic guidance and the ability to recover.

The Ancient Greeks considered the soul (or psyche) to be a moving dynamic force capable of being influenced not only to induce disease, but also to restore harmony. Human problems, and the physical manifestations of illness, were viewed essentially as spiritual in nature; literally as 'psychopathology' (Graham, 1999). The Greeks were keen observers of feelings and moods, and emotional purging and laughter were viewed as highly therapeutic. Mythology and Greek theatre were also considered useful and necessary, often used to explain the meaning of otherwise difficult concepts, and to invoke and induce intense emotional responses. Greek philosophers during this time certainly considered man's health to lie centrally within the remit of their thinking.

"The cure of the part should not be attempted without treatment of the whole" - Plato

In essence the early Greeks believed the key to maintaining good health lay in achieving a balance between the spiritual, and the physical elements of life. To the Greeks of this period, however, the Gods were still deemed influential, and the Greek temple priests continued to practice a great deal of the ancient knowledge inherited from the Egyptians in their own particular form of medicine.

Pythagorean Mathematics and Rational Medicine

During the sixth century BC the influence of Pythagorean philosophy marked the beginning of mathematics and coding and represents the birth of modern science and linear thinking. Pythagorean theory influenced Western thinking tremendously simply because mathematics sits at the core of the concepts of exact and measurable truths.

"Greek medicine, generally, formed the basis of Western medical theory until the nineteenth century and Greek medical deontology still exercises a powerful influence upon medical ethics to the present day." (Longrigg, 1993).

Within the field of medicine the first indication of the practice of human dissection occurred during the fifth century BC, representing the emergence of the scientific concepts of exploration, analysis, measurement and standardisation in health and medicine.

Hippocrates

During the 5th century BC, Hippocrates, commonly regarded as the father of modern medicine, introduced his medical *'theory of four humors and temperaments'*. According to Hippocrates physical disorders could be viewed as conditions of disharmony existing in the humors of the body. Hippocrates believed the individual could be affected by many factors, including thoughts and emotions, behaviours, climate, excessive or too little physical activity, water quality, and even a lack of sunlight. Hippocrates believed healing could take place when equilibrium was restored in both the psychology, and the internal and external environment of the individual. He stated treatment should only occur after consideration of attitude, environmental influences and natural remedies, and placed worth on the individual's ability to self heal given favourable conditions. The role of physician according to Hippocrates was therefore one of serving natural laws.

Parmenides

During the mid 5th century BC the Greek philosopher Parmenides proposed physical matter was an indestructible substance made up of tiny dead particles he coined atoms. The movement of these atoms was assumed by the ancient

Greeks to originate from the spiritual, although the matter itself was viewed as somehow different and separate. Philosophers of the time now began to turn their attention away from the subject of considering physical matter and how it might be connected to human life, and began instead to lean towards more existential, spiritual and ethical considerations. Scientific thinking would now take responsibility for dissecting and measuring the nature of universal physical matter, including the human body.

Christianity and the Middle Ages

The emergence of Christianity and its subsequent spread across Western Europe delivered an enormous blow to man's innate, ancient connection with his own personal energetic power and intuition. Man began to be guided towards a belief in one omnipotent God, and the church took authority on his behalf. Scientists throughout the middle-ages, under the watchful eye of the Christian Church, continued to attempt to explain the existence of God, and the nature of universe, using a standardized framework drawn from the concepts of Greek scientific reasoning. During this time a real and definite attempt was made by the Church to destroy any movement, group or individual still ingrained with any belief system associated with ancient, esoteric knowledge. The healers of the day were those infused with the secrets of oral medicinal folk traditions; commonly referred to as witches during the middle-ages. Evidence stemming from witch trials dating to the time suggests indeed a great deal of the knowledge possessed by these often female healers might be viewed as essentially shamanic in origin.

Scientific Milestones

It was Copernicus (1473-1543) who first proposed the notion that the planets circled the sun, and in doing so challenged Church teachings stating the earth lay at the centre of the universe. The laws of planetary motion discovered by Kepler (1571-1630) further challenged the deeply established religious view, and the final proof was delivered by Galileo (1564-1642) when he demonstrated the earth did indeed revolve around the sun. Collectively this marked a time of huge collision and separation between science and religion. Within the realm of health and medicine this period in history also sparked the emergence of what we recognise today as modern medicine. In 1543, Andreas Vesalius published an important human anatomy book. In 1628, William Harvey published his research on the circulation of blood in the body, and finally the microscope, an enormously important technological advancement in medicine, was invented in 1670 by Anton van Leeuwenhoek.

Newton's Influence

Isaac Newton (1643-1727) believed the universe to be a three-dimensional space. An immovable, constant, unchangeable place existing entirely independently of the material objects contained within. According to Newton, changes in the physical world existed in a separate dimension of time, which absolute in nature, flowed in a linear sequence. Newton proposed small particles existed in this place, and believed gravity to be the force which explained the movement of the particles. Consequently scientific thinking now began to consider the universe, and the very essence of nature itself, as following an unquestionable mechanistic model, with every component of life considered explainable by a cosmic set of fixed rules, governed by absolute mathematical laws and equations.

The Separation of Body and Mind

By the nineteenth century science had become so entrenched in a Newtons' mechanistic view of the universe, the concept of God had almost become obsolete. The advent of modern physics, and a growing insistence within the scientific world that all things should be universally agreed upon as objective, physical and factual, left the field of psychology with a quite a dilemma. Traditionally known for embracing the concepts of consciousness, senses and feelings; elements which ultimately could never be measured objectively, yet still anxious to be recognised and listed as a scientific endeavour, the field of psychology chose to turn away from the study of human emotion and psyche and instead began to concentrate on the objective study of human behaviour (Graham, 1999). Science and medicine now began to view the physical elements of the individual as existing entirely separately from the mind and psyche. The diagnosis and treatment of disease and illness within Western medicine has been considered in this somewhat fragmented context since.

It was the publishing of Albert Einstein's Special Theory of Relativity in 1905, closely followed by Rutherford's historic splitting of the atom in 1909, that finally pulled apart the by now established mechanical, clockwork Newtonian view of the world. According to Einstein time and space are ultimately connected, and four dimensional in essence. Whereas previously time was considered as fixed and linear, Einstein's theory states time is dynamic, able to stretch and move, and absolutely and intrinsically linked to space, and indeed, to the matter contained within.

Summary

It would appear over time individuals have become increasingly disconnected from their own personal experience and almost entirely passive regarding their health-care. Conversely science, medicine, doctors and other healthcare workers have been encouraged to adopt a professional stance of detached authority and assumed superior knowledge. The complex physiological and emotional relationships present within the human body were unfortunately initially judged by early science as deserving of no place in fact, or the absolute, instead dismissed almost entirely in favour of a mathematical understanding of man. Science and the medical profession have become the modern day Gods, and human individuals are now more detached from their own existence and personal responsibility than they have been in perhaps many thousands of years.

"The more specialised doctors become, the more they know about a body part or organ and the less they tend to understand the human being in whom that part or organ resides." (Mate, 2003).

The separation of mind and body, and indeed man from his wider experiencing unfortunately dictates man can never truly be perceived, measured, or treated as a whole. As practitioners of reflexology, or indeed any holistic modality, it seems crucial as we move into the future we strive to retain a blend of practice retaining a truly holistic, multi-dimensional essence. Twentieth century physics suggests a basic oneness exists within our universe. These up to date scientific principles suggest we inhabit a far more complex and interactive universe than could ever have been imagined. Perhaps in time we might come to increasingly accept this concept also applies in the consideration of human health.

"A fundamental problem facing contemporary medicine is that of reconciling ordinary descriptions of bodies, health and disease with the idea that the universe and everything in it is an inseparable entity." (Graham, 1999)

Encouragingly the scientific field of psychoneuroimmunology (PNI); a relatively young branch of research established during the early 1980s, offers both western medical, and holistic researchers alike, a scientific framework from which to better understand the complex interactions between the mind, brain, and wider body. What the Shamans, Ancients, and healers of the Middle Ages might have referred to as *personal power*, today we call the *autonomous, conscious self*.

Perhaps one thing reflexologists do very well is to help clients to reconnect with their personal power, through interpersonal touch, support, encouragement, and advice? Perhaps too, within modern day complementary therapies, exist many threads connecting our holistic art forms to the health philosophies of the far distant past?

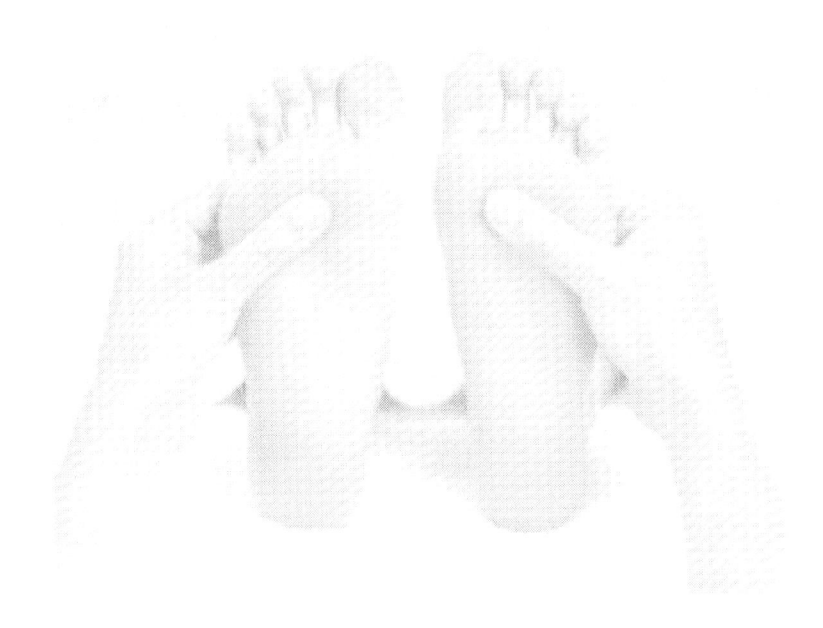

Relational Reflexology

Reflexology? That's All About the Feet, Right?

"Thank you for your knowledge and skills, your patience, your dedication, keeping me going when I'd had enough, putting up with my moaning, answering my questions, no matter how silly, involving me in decisions, teaching me to keep calm and relaxed, being understanding and providing support, believing in me, helping to make dreams come true."

- Rachael - A Reflexology Client

As professional reflexology practitioners we are indeed fortunate to be in a position to offer both the time and environment required to build effective therapeutic relationships with our clients. Indeed, the quality of the therapeutic relationship formed between an attentive reflexologist and their client can perhaps be likened to no other occurring in the field of complementary therapies. The modality, practiced face to face, and involving the powerful medium of touch might be viewed as a deeply intimate, complementary practice. The transformative power contained within the reflexology relationship has the potential to reach far beyond the boundaries of an hour long session of touch, pressure and relaxation. In our busy time limited world, certainly from the perspective of the anxious client, the beneficial effects of being held in a safe therapeutic relationship, whilst being touched, supported, educated, and encouraged should not perhaps be underestimated.

Looking more closely at the experience of my own client it seems Rachel rated *knowledge*, *skills* and *support* as being of value, as well as mentioning *patience, a listening ear* and feelings of being *involved* and *encouraged*.

It would seem Rachel was able not only to *receive* the physical application of reflexology, but also to *perceive* - and therefore potentially react to - some form of emotional support stemming from the reflexology relationship.

Of course many reflexology exchanges are also impacting clients sense of well-being multi-dimensionally, within the clients physical realm (through touch and pressure), and the clients emotional and intellectual **realms** (through support and learning). Perhaps reflexology is indeed a complementary modality perfectly packaged to meet the complex multi-dimensional phenomenology of many presenting clients?

Understanding Phenomenology

Phenomenology is in essence the study of individual perception and consciousness. The phenomenological approach refers to a particular set of perspectives, or methodologies, used to carry out **qualitative** research investigations. Phenomenological questioning originated in response to the scientific stance related to considering only that assessed to be objective and measurable. Phenomenology is therefore concerned with attempting to unfold dimensions of human experience, through exploring how individuals experience within their unique world.

Phenomenological thinking states:

- No perception can be entirely objective.

- Every perception owes as much to the mentality of the perceiver, as it does to the structure of the object.

- A great deal of human experience is non-repeatable and so virtually unmeasurable.

A phenomenological enquiry might attempt to explore:

- What is distinct in each person's experience?

- What is common to the experience of certain groups of people who have shared the same events, or circumstances?

Why is it important to understand about relational concepts?

It might be easy momentarily to forget as we reflect on these positive words that Rachel initially made contact as an emotionally vulnerable client. Undoubtedly, dealing with emotional content is an ethically delicate and challenging matter, and one requiring some level of considered thought. However, it is also worth remembering that dealing with emotional content is an integral part of the human experience, and therefore - for most people - a shared experience.

It may be that individuals sometimes opt to engage in complementary therapies (such as reflexology), because they view the modality as less authoritative, or clinically formal. This may also mean clients choose to view their complementary practitioner in a less authoritative manner; preferring to consider the practitioner as more of a *helper*, or perhaps simply as *someone who cares*. Certainly, the lack of pre-defined official boundaries within our reflexology consulting rooms, perhaps of the kind more commonly associated with traditional health-care professionals, means client emotional disclosure can be a relatively common occurrence within many reflexology exchanges.

If we can openly acknowledge clients are disclosing their emotions to their reflexologists, and that *we*, as practitioners of reflexology, seem perfectly willing to listen, the next step is to ensure the highest standard of relational skills in practice. Perhaps the single most important ethical challenge our profession currently faces is how to ensure reflexology practitioners are relating safely with emotionally vulnerable clients?

As practitioners of course, we alone are responsible for the standards we set within our own individual practice - anyone for a beginners counselling course?

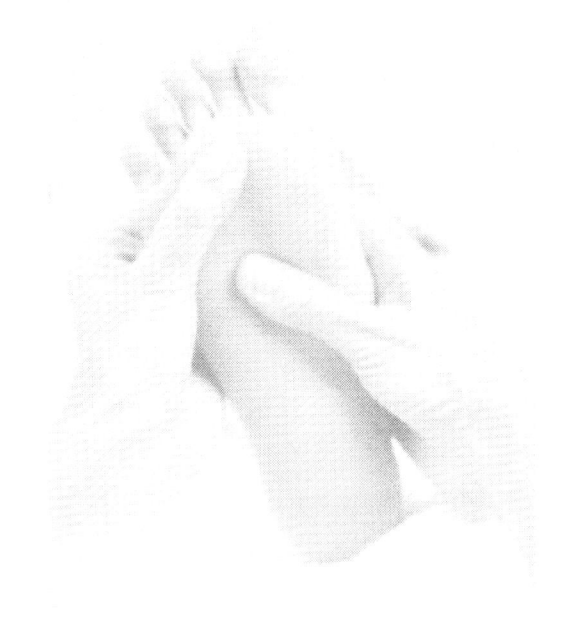

Relational Reflexology

Reflexology Flavours

"Many paths lead from the foot of the mountain, but at the peak we all gaze at the same single bright moon."

- Ikkyu

My personal form of practice in reflexology is heavily influenced by the principles of Traditional Chinese Medicine - principally because I completed my first auricular acupuncture course mid-way through my reflexology training. At the time I can recall feeling relieved to be introduced to a health philosophy where emotional states remained intact. I can also recall completing a case study with a client who presented with the most inflexible feet, coupled with deep stagnation/heavy granular deposits across the lung reflex area. This client reported no respiratory disorder. Those familiar with TCM will be aware of the close association between lung energy, over thinking, deep stress, grief, and anxiety. The client in question was a deeply stressed individual, and fairly uncomfortable with emotion. The TCM link made more sense to me. *I could work with that!*

I don't know a great deal about other reflexology theories if I'm honest. I found a rationale that worked for me, and pretty much remained faithful to it. I did choose to develop my relational skills further and trained as a person-centred counsellor. I also worked to improve my anatomy and physiology knowledge, so as to better understand the clinical conditions clients presented with. My client base consists mostly of sub-fertility, chronic anxiety and migraine clients, and so perhaps unsurprisingly I have come to find myself reasonably knowledgable about the endocrine and reproductive systems, in addition to the bodies stress responses. I know next to nothing about working with brain injured clients, or about work in a hospice. I have only once treated a client with cancer, and I know very little about MS, or a host of other health conditions I have not yet encountered. As a reflexologist I am constructed of many parts and I clearly have gaps in my knowledge. I certainly do not profess to be an all knowing healer. I have been influenced by my initial reflexology **training**, my choice of continuing professional development (**CPD**), my real therapeutic practice and **experience**, and of course, my **personality**

What really seems important is *how* we utilise the knowledge we gain (from any reflexology theoretical standpoint), and that the information is used appropriately and reflectively with clients. Through sharing our knowledge wisely we are far more able to promote the concepts of autonomy, and self directed client change. The unique library of information and experience each individual practitioner gathers serves to lift us from the place of fledging reflexologist - *trying desperately to recall where the thyroid reflex is situated* - to a place where we're more able to engage with our clients confidently and therapeutically. We are now able to engage with the *whole* person, not just the feet.

As we each walk our unique reflexology path undoubtedly we must carry with us high professional standards, good levels of appropriate knowledge, robust ethics, and a strong inner supervisor, but clearly the reflexology path is likely to differ for us all. I have chosen to extend my skills package in a particular way, and to adopt a particular rationale for my reflexology practice, but it is not the *only* way. I am entirely unique, and so too my particular flavour of therapy is unique. What we have in common certainly is our love of reflexology, and a deep desire to help others.

Reflexology – A Therapeutic Art Form
Not a Procedure

"Ours is a society that has perfected its means, yet neglected its meaning."

- Albert Einstein

What exactly is Reflexology? At first glance this might seem a relatively simple question to answer. Peer a little deeper however, and the question is actually much more complex. Undoubtedly, this is an important question, and one worth some considerable reflection by both individual reflexology practitioners, and indeed our wider therapeutic community. Reflexology has been defined by the the Department of Health (UK) as:

"Application of pressure to the hands and feet to promote well-being."

Recently, the Reflexology in Europe Network (RIEN) agreed upon their working definition of reflexology:

"Reflexology deals with the principle that there are reflex areas on the feet that correspond with different parts of the body and it is a method that affects these reflex areas to attain wellbeing."

Encouragingly in recent years our therapeutic modality has started to collate a small body of favourable valid clinical research. Understanding for example, the specific mechanics of action relating to reflexology is indeed an important and utterly worthwhile endeavour. Each new piece of research, no matter how small, either suggesting or better demonstrating any specific physiological mechanics, undoubtedly helps to strengthen the reputation of the modality, and promote a wider understanding of any potential therapeutic worth.

It is also worth remembering that one of the reasons the modality has been able to attract higher levels of clinical research interest is simply because the general public keep choosing to utilise reflexology. It is undoubtedly our client's positive reaction to reflexology, across many decades; *their* antidotal evidence and *their* personal recommendations, in addition to the observations of experienced practitioners that enabled the modality to reach a place now deemed worthy of more in-depth clinical research and investigation. The previous heavy lean in research towards examining the mechanics of action using *sham* reflexology points for example, means the modality has the unfortunate tendency to be viewed from a somewhat limited perspective; that being one of only examining the relationship between the potential reflex points and any associated specific impact. That said, from a practitioner standpoint it is entirely encouraging and affirming to read of any positive research emerging.

One such recent Japanese study (Naoki et al, 2013), looked at the effects of using specific reflexology stimulation to the eye reflex point/area utilising fMRI to record brain activity in recipients. The study demonstrated:

"a robust relationship exists between neural processing of somatosensory percepts for reflexological stimulation and the tactile sensation of a specific reflex area in the left middle postcentral gyrus, the area to which tactile sensation to the face projects, as well as in the postcentral gyrus contralateral foot representation area."

and that:

"This activity was not affected by pseudo information."

So here we have some pretty wonderful positive research. No conjecture, no opinion, just good solid scientific fact. The nature of the research, whilst limited by construct and pre-defined question, is precisely the kind of positive clinical enquiry required to demonstrate the underlying principles of reflexology. Does this Japanese research help to explain what reflexology really is? The research certainly tells us more about what happens when we stimulate feet through touch and pressure. It also clearly helps to back up the hypothesis stating there are areas on the feet which correspond to certain parts of the body, but does the study help to explain why so many people report such positive reactions to reflexology, or to explain the dynamics of what might be occurring within the confines of a practitioner's therapy room? A realistic and balanced answer to these questions is clearly - *only in part*. What this research fails to tell us is how any neurological activity might be affecting the eye more specifically, nor does this type of research help us to examine the wider aspects of a therapeutic reflexology encounter. Even in those instances where practitioners choose to carry out reflexology sessions in complete silence, fuller and more realistic research parameters would need to consider:

The **wider physiological effects of touch** on the mind, brain, and body - blood pressure, heart rate - the effects of touch on cortisone and adrenaline levels - the release of endorphins, neuropeptides, serotonin and dopamine.

Client intention: Simply picking up the phone and attending for reflexology might be considered as demonstrating positive mental intention. This can promote both a positive psychological and physiological response

Internal emotional responses: Even during reflexology performed in silence client's are often not fully asleep, but more in a deeply relaxed, potentially internally reflective state. These individual subjective, psychologically rooted processes are extremely difficult, if not impossible, to quantify within a classic scientific paradigm.

The therapeutic relationship: Even on a basic level the consultation period is likely to be impacting therapeutic outcomes primarily because of the focus of attention being placed on client experience and past history.

Increased existential thinking: Even on a very basic level practitioners often encourage client self care towards the end of the reflexology session; rest, water, avoiding stimulants etc.

Each new piece of clinical research, new advanced technique, or theory of application presented to practitioners represents a small piece of much more complex jigsaw. It is important we are able to remain open and objective as we move forward in attempting to defining reflexology more fully. We should strive to encompass a wholly holistic overview otherwise we may be in danger of becoming represented by a medically defined representation of the whole reflexology package.

Leaning too heavily towards understanding the exact mechanics of a reflexology encounter from a solely quantifiable stand-point might be akin to trying to understand the taste and texture of a chocolate cake through describing its molecular structure. Whilst it might be useful to know how it is constructed, perhaps it's the taste that really counts.

The flourishing scientific field of psychoneuroimmunology is encouragingly bringing together those previously fragmented medical, psychological, and sociological disciplines. In the future this more complex multi-dimensional approach to understanding human health will undoubtedly require a more complex holistic and kaleidoscopic form of research enquiry. An enquiry also better suited to exploring the multi-dimensional phenomenology of the reflexology package.

I am a reflexologist. I might define this personally by stating; *I engage therapeutically with people using reflexology'*, and not; *'I work with peoples feet'*. I am a therapist and my modality is a therapeutic art form, not a procedure. I hope as we move into the future we never lose sight of that.

Verbal Communication and Client Emotional Disclosure Practitioner Survey Findings

The survey was an informal existential enquiry designed to explore the attitudes of professional practitioners regarding verbal communication and client emotional disclosure within their reflexology practice.

The survey findings suggest verbal communications (instructional, supportive, or explanatory) to be fairly common in reflexology.

The findings also suggest the presence of client emotional content to be fairly common in reflexology, with many participants considering emotional content as a simply naturally occurring phenomenon in reflexology.

Findings also suggest professional practitioners have a good understanding of professional concepts related to both competency boundaries, and professional referral within reflexology. The survey was constructed of six multiple choice questions, with space provided for additional participant comments. The survey required no identifying participant information.

Survey Method and Participants

The survey was live and accessible for one week and offered to professional reflexology practitioners via social networking reflexology groups on both Facebook and Twitter. Survey data was shared with Tracey Smith - Reflexology and Research Manager, Association of Reflexologists, UK, to encourage transparency and reduce bias.

Survey Response

The survey returned **142** completed responses, with **495** comments from practitioners in **16** countries.

- UK – **69%** (98)
- United States – **11%** (15)
- Ireland – **5%** (7)
- Canada – **3%** (4)
- New Zealand – **2%** (3)
- Norway, Greece, France, Australia - **1%** each (2)
- Portugal, Romania, Malta, India, Spain, Hungary, Jordan – **1%** each (1)

Survey Coding

Due to the high number of written comments existing in the survey data (**495**) the **Duquesne method** was chosen to evaluate the information. The Duquesne method is a qualitative research tool associated specifically with **phenomenological research**. The procedures for collating information in this manner were first written about within a social science context by Colaizzi (1978), then Bullington and Karlsson (1984), Wertz (1984), Hycner (1985), Polkinghorne (1989) and Moustakas (1994).

The ultimate research goal associated with this phenomenological approach is *'to elucidate the essence of the phenomenon being studied, as it exists in participants' concrete experience'* (McLoud, 2001). The researcher is therefore attempting to identify central *themes* or *meanings* implicit in the statements of the participants, before attempting to integrate these meanings into a single description of any phenomenon.

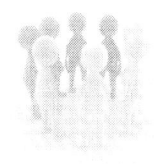

Question One

Do you ever talk/chat with your clients during a reflexology session?

[142 responses (0 skips) and 104 individual comments]

- It depends on the individual client – **73.5%** (107)
- Yes, I often chat with my clients – **15.49%** (22)
- Yes, but only ever during the consultation period – **4.93%** (7)
- No, I would never encourage talking during a session – **4.23%** (6)

Question One Themes – *'Client Leads'*

Q 1. comments are mostly associated with the concept of remaining respectful of the clients choice in how they use the therapeutic reflexology space. The survey suggests many practitioners seem content to engage in verbal exchanges if initiated by the client. Comments suggest participants try to focus on the clients presenting needs, and adapt to verbal interaction were necessary.

Comments:

- "I let the client decide, it's their time"
- "You can gauge if a client wants to relax, or if they want to chat. I go with the flow"
- "It should be client led for optimum effectiveness"
- "I am led by the client"
- "Some clients need to chat so I adapt my treatments accordingly"
- "Some people want to chat, others don't. I let the client lead the way"

- "I am always listening and reading between the lines to see what the client wants and what they need. It's a dance."

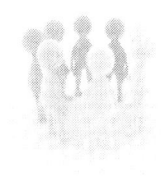

Question Two

Do you provide any form of interpretation to your reflexology clients? For example to help explain why a certain point might feel painful, or tender?

[127 responses (15 skips) and 98 individual comments]

- Yes, I always attempt to give an interpretation to clients – **88%** (112)
- No, I never attempt to offer an interpretation – **12%** (15)

Question Two Themes – *'Clients Often Want to Know but I Don't Diagnose*

Three interrelated themes emerged from the comments relating to Q 2. Those themes are respectively connected to interpretation being offered when requested by the client, the nature of those interpretations, and finally, the existence of a transparent practitioner consciousness relating to the concept of avoiding diagnosis in reflexology.

Participant comments seem to suggest that whilst interpretation in some form is frequently occurring within reflexology exchanges, many of these interpretations are manifesting as a result of client enquiries, or responses to pain.

Additionally, comments seem to suggest the existence of a clear attentiveness towards avoiding interactions, or conversations that may potentially be interpreted by the client diagnostically. The survey suggests interpretations are therefore often delivered multi-theoretically, i.e. possible direct foot issues, foot map associations, cross reflex associations, TCM associations, etc. Offering such conscious multi-theoretical interpretations seems to ensure practitioners avoid making definite statements.

Comments:

- "I interpret in general terms according to the client's level of interest"
- "Yes if a point is painful and they ask about it I give a few different interpretations so it's not a definite truth, but instead a little insight"
- "I like to inform clients that there are different interpretations for certain areas & this often leads to more in depth conversations"
- "Yes, because most clients ask "why is this area tender." Then I will answer"
- "If I can interpret it into a physical or emotional, or both, I offer this up as to why the area may be painful. Then the client can elaborate if they want to. I never diagnose, or say this IS what it is .."
- "I explain which reflex point they are feeling. I don't offer a diagnosis"
- "I keep the information very general, simply stating that they may be a little out of balance in the corresponding part of the body, or referred part of the body, or even say it may be a problem with the foot"
- "Very careful not to scare, but share thoughts on possibilities for the discomfort"
- "Only when they ask will I then interpret, but stating different opinions of various schools of thought (reflexology, TCM, emotions, etc). I try not to produce nocebo"
- "Not always – but I find most clients want to know "what have you found" and I explain this as a tension in a certain area, they then ask what reflex it is and then some do ask what I think it mean – to which I say I can never claim to diagnose"

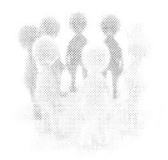

Question Three

How do you feel about the presence of client emotional content in your therapy room?

[139 responses (3 skips) and 84 individual comments]

- I feel confident in my ability to deal with client emotional content in my therapy room - 81.29% (113)
- I am fine with the presence of client emotional content in my therapy room, but don't always feel confident in my relating skills - 13.67% (19)
- I feel very uncomfortable with the presence of client emotional content in my therapy room – 5.04% (7)
- I try very hard not to encourage the disclosure of client emotional content in my therapy room – 0%

Question Three Themes – *'Reflexology and Emotion'*

The first theme emerging from Q 3. relates to the participants wider intellectual definition of reflexology: specifically that many practitioners acknowledge a close association existing between the physical modality, and the presence, or release of, client emotional content.

Comments:

- "It goes without saying there will be some emotional clearing with a treatment"
- "The physical self and emotional self are after all interconnected"

- "A therapist's ability to be open to a client's emotional needs is one of the core benefits of any kind of therapy"
- "No one comes in the door without emotion"
- "(Emotional release) is an important part of the treatment"
- "I believe the physical act of reflexology and listening to emotive subjects goes hand in hand"
- "Emotions are an intrinsic part of the holistic approach to health"
- "(Emotion) is part of reflexology"
- #"I find that emotional and physical problems are connected"

Question Three Themes - *'Professional Boundaries and Referral'*

The second theme relates to a wide acknowledgement of professional concepts in the comments, for example, subjects such as boundaries and limitations existing within the practitioner's professional remit are mentioned, as well as the concept of professional referral.

Additionally, some reference was made to prior, or potentially required, relational/emotional concept training.

Comments:

- "I know my limits and boundaries"
- "I am mindful of my professional boundaries"
- "Sometimes I feel I should do a counselling course"
- "Sometimes I'm unsure how to help"
- "I'm very happy to recommend that professional help may be necessary"
- "If the client needs counselling or referring – I would do so"
- "(In a multidisciplinary team) you know that you have the support and further services to refer a client if you need to"
- "I have experience of emotional/psychological issues from a previous career"
- "My previous work (nursing) taught me the skill of listening"

- "(I've) worked for a helpline charity"

Question Three Themes - *'Intention and Listening'*

The third theme relates to the practitioners general intention within the reflexology environment. Participants made heavy mention of the concept of listening within this context.

Comments:

- "I encourage (clients) to be open and let them know their information will be treated as confidential"
- "I consider it as an honour and privilege when a client opens up to me about their issues"
- "It's all about creating a space for (clients) to release what they need to release"
- "I have a lot to offer, a lot of experience to draw on"
- "I don't feel the need to offer advice or to take a stance on any given situation, but feel that my 'being there' as an outsider can prove very helpful"
- "I offer an open ear and sometimes that's enough for the client"
- "We are there to listen"
- "If a client feels confident enough in me to want to discuss their feelings them that is fine by me"
- "Sometimes a client is happy to talk and I just sit and listen"
- "Listening is a part of the professional service"

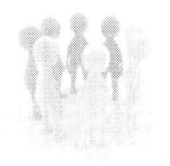

Question Four

In which setting do you normally work as a reflexologist?

[141 responses (1 skip) and 68 individual comments]

- Private Practice - **80%** (113)
- A Clinical/Medical Type Setting – **11%** (16)
- A Spa/Beauty Type Setting - **6%** (8)
- A Hospice Type Setting – **3%** (4)

Question Four Themes – *'In Private Practice'*

Q.4. comments mostly verified the information provided in the associated multiple choice questions. Perhaps the most interesting theme to emerge from this question relates to the heavy lean in responses from practitioners in private practice; this perhaps mirroring generally the existing ratio of clinically based/privately practicing reflexologists? This small, informal survey perhaps provides us with an interesting interpretation of how reflexology is practiced more generally, and therefore also experienced by the general public.

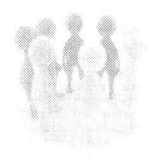

Question Five

Reflexology equates to what % of your weekly work?

[140 responses (2 skips) and 64 individual comments]

- Reflexology equates to 50-75% of my client base – 37.14% (52)
- I practice reflexology exclusively – 35.71% (50)
- Reflexology equates to less than 25% of my client base – 14.29% (20)
- Reflexology equates to 25-50% of my client base – 12.86% (18)

Question Five Themes

Q 5. comments mostly verified the information provided in the multiple choice question. Comments in the section demonstrated a mix of full-time and part-time therapists – some practitioners retaining part-time employment outside of their reflexology practice, whilst another significant group practiced reflexology alongside an additional therapeutic modality.

Comments:

- "I practice other therapies e.g. Aromatherapy/Massage etc"
- "50% practice nurse, 50% reflexology"
- "I am also a qualified acupuncturist and combine the 2 treatments very nicely"
- "I have an additional part-time job"

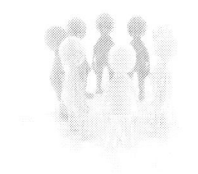

Question Six

Do you offer advice to your clients regarding diet, exercise, or relaxation techniques etc?

[140 responses (2 skips) and 77 individual comments]

- Yes, I give general advice regarding water, increased rest periods etc – **57.86%** (81)
- Yes, I give specific advice to each client – **40%** (56)
- No, I never give advice – **2.14%** (4)

Question Six Themes – *"I Give Advice – But I Know My Boundaries"*

Overall two themes emerged from Q.6. comments. Comments mostly made reference to any advice as offered specific to client needs. The comments suggest whilst the advice is general in essence, it can cover a broad spectrum of subjects depending on the individual client, and might include; increasing mobility, cutting back on detrimental food types, increasing periods of self care, hydration, and teaching relaxation techniques. A large group of participants also made reference to working within professional competencies with regards to giving advice, and appeared mindful of utilising professional referral.

Comments:

- *"I offer common sense advice: meditate if stressed, have me time, etc"*
- *"I also teach meditation techniques for relaxation etc"*
- *"They all get an aftercare sheet, if they are having a problem I show them on their hands – they can do it themselves"*

- "It depends in client what I say and again it's more if they ask. I am qualified in lots if therapies and have lots of experience and knowledge beyond reflexology. I always lead by the client though"
- "I give general advice and also more specific advice in areas in which I am qualified"
- "I share that I know a little about a lot and often guide them to another professional in the field of health if need be"

Summary

- The survey findings suggest many professional reflexology practitioners are engaging verbally on some level with their clients; either on an instructional (advice), supportive (listening and reflection) or explanatory (interpretation) level, or a combination of the three. Much of that interaction appears to be client led.

- The survey also suggests the presence of client emotional disclosure/release is considered by many participants as somewhere between desirable and expected.

- Encouragingly, the vast majority of respondents made unprompted acknowledgment of their attentiveness towards professional boundaries, and of utilising professional referral, where necessary.

- The survey perhaps also interestingly demonstrates how much power a client holds in their freedom to utilise the reflexology space as they wish. Reflexology practitioners seem willing and open to accept the multi-dimensional nature of many clients; content to hold the body, whilst accommodating any accompanying emotions. Reflexologists seem to accept their clients with hands outstretched, and ears wide open, ready to touch, listen, and support.

Future Recommendations

1. In order to promote a more objective multi-dimensional interpretation of the reflexology package clearly more formal research is required to assess the potential impact of the client/practitioner relationship.
2. Existing practitioners can choose to actively enhance their knowledge of therapeutic relational skills.
3. Professional training schools can choose to widen the perimeters of their course syllabus to incorporate modules related to therapeutic relational skills.
4. Practitioners with duel training (reflexology/counselling) might consider constructing good quality CPD courses addressing these important concepts.

Researchers' Comments - *The Middle Place – The Listening Place*

"The growth of complementary therapies to meet demand is unequivocal. Psychological trauma is at its most concentrated; we are suffering from overload and we need a safe space in which we may tell our story." (March-Smith, 2005)

There is a place within the concept of relating – a place deeper than general associating - but not quite the probing exploration associated with counselling and psychotherapy; that place involves **active listening**. Reflexologists certainly seem to be adept at offering a space in which clients choose to be heard.

This middle place - *the listening place* – is already acknowledged with our wider society as highly valuable and required. Well known organisations here in the UK, such as the Samaritans, Child Line, St John Ambulance, and Victim Support provide a listening service to members of the general public. Additionally, there any many other, community based projects and support charities offering similar listening services. The greater majority of these organisations require their volunteers to engage in at least some basic relational and boundary skills training.

If we are to begin to fully champion and acknowledge the potential multi-dimensional impact of the reflexology package, and therefore start to focus more fully on the impact of the relationship between the client and the practitioner, in the future, as a CAM industry we might fare well from introducing relational skills into our training programmes.

"Very little is taught about the therapeutic relationship, its importance and how to create effective ones, on complementary therapy trainings. Research shows that the most important factor in a successful psychotherapy treatment is the relationship between the therapist and the client, not the school or model of counselling used. If these findings are translatable to complementary therapy then it could mean that the relationship with an individual CAM practitioner is as important as the therapy she or he practices." (Fox, 2008)

Research suggests many therapists are drawn to our type of profession process innate natural relating skills, and a deep desire to help others. Is that quite enough in this modern world of standardisation and defined boundaries? Should we, like other listening services, begin to absorb basic relating concepts into our training?

Perhaps the time has come for the wider reflexology industry to start to highlight the often intimate interactions between practitioner and client, and champion our modality in its full multi-dimensional wonder? Perhaps also the time has come for professional practitioners to begin to become attentive during some of their professional development time to the relating side of their reflexology practice? It is after all, mind, body, spirit.

A Place for Love in Reflexology?

He whom love touches not walks in darkness."

- Plato

Is there a place for love in the reflexology exchange? Is love a relevant subject? Should we draw attention to the concept? Does it possess any measurable, clinical value? As our wider therapeutic modality moves forward in attempting to define a more precise representation of the art of reflexology these are questions certainly perhaps worth further consideration.

In other therapeutic disciplines where forms of therapeutic love can be present, for example, talking therapies and nursing, the concept of love existing in therapeutic relationships can often be intellectually challenging, as practitioners find they grapple with complicated professional boundary issues. For many professional reflexologists, however, the concept of love existing in our practice might be a slightly less challenging consideration? Often a practitioner's knowledge relating to energy work, or mediation practices, such as reiki, yoga, and mindfulness concepts can have the tendency to promote a wider intellectual definition of the word *love*. Additionally, the concepts of love (*honour*) and intention (*action*) are often intertwined for many CAM practitioners.

For the purpose of this article the term 'love' is defined as non-romantic, non-sexual, and non-power based within the context of therapeutic encounters.

"Love is a tricky word to use in a therapeutic context. It's used almost exclusively in popular culture to mean falling in love, or as a synonym for sex, and all the other variants like maternal love, filial love, love for one's fellow human beings, or spiritual love have less of a place in common currency." (Fox, 2008)

Certainly many of our reflexology clients benefit from clear boundaries, guidance, encouragement, information, honesty and integrity; each one in their own way, perhaps an extension of therapeutic love, exemplified as the loving parent offers care to a troubled or injured child or adolescent?

What other qualities are professional reflexology practitioners attempting to demonstrate to their clients?

- **Care?**

- **Tenderness?**

- **Compassion?**

- **Attention?**

- **Focus?**

Perhaps is it possible these essentially personal practitioner qualities also represent some form of therapeutic based love displaying in the reflexology relationship? How might we better define this therapeutic found love, and is it actually required, or valuable within a reflexology context? Isn't it enough just to work the feet well, and sufficiently?

Therapeutic type love is perhaps in essence a representation of love, appreciation, and acceptance for the unique individual. Carl Rogers (1951), referred to this type of therapeutic love as unconditional positive regard.

Unconditional Positive Regard

The client feels valued and accepted as they are: the practitioner may not approve of the client's actions, but the practitioner does wholly approve of the client.

What does it mean to unconditionally regard a person? To find unconditional acceptance for every client certainly isn't always easy. Ideally, UPR develops as a part of a practitioner's life philosophy, or personal value system. Perhaps it is best summed up as a way of finding respect for the value of every human being. UPR requires us to find genuine warmth and acceptance for each of our clients. No matter how good a person we might think we are, or how charitable we might try to be, every individual is judgemental to some degree. Connecting through our inner judgements to reach the innate worth and value of an individual is to develop unconditional positive regard.

Developing a more non-judgemental attitude can certainly help to prevent blocks from forming within the therapeutic relationship. It can certainly be easy to disagree with the life choices of a individual, but that disapproval should never be allowed to hinder the fostering of genuine warmth and care within the relationship. Nourishing the concept of UPR helps us therefore to better demonstrate to our clients that they are wholly valued and accepted, just as they are.

Love in Human Relating

"Love is the only way to grasp another human being in the innermost core of his personality. No one can become aware of the very essence of another human being unless he loves him." - Viktor Frankl

Undoubtedly every day professional reflexology practitioners are attempting to love and care for their clients; touching, encouraging and nourishing, as a parent might love and nourish the potential in the child. Reflexologists clearly display many forms of care in their therapeutic interactions, often through their very being, their real presence, as they hold, touch, encourage, and try to make safe their clients.

How important is this *connection* in the work we undertake with clients?

Does our *intention* really matter?

Love Communicated Through Touch

"Touch, along with other forms of non-verbal expression (gestures, facial expressions etc), is a language, a means of communication." (Smith et al, 1998)

Scientific research provides us with a better understanding of the beneficial effects of touch on the human body. The skin is the largest organ in the human body, and loaded with receptors connected to touch, pain, temperature and pressure.

"Nourishing physical touch is in fact one of the most significant factors influencing growth." (Williams et al, 2011)

Touch is acknowledged as an important element of many human interactions. Appropriate touch for example is considered as absolutely necessary to children, both psychologically and developmentally. Touch has been identified in many studies as promoting feelings of reassurance, and affirmation of existence.

"Touch is an important part of being human, a way in which our consciousness is redrawn into our physical being, and our very existence confirmed" (Jourard, 1966)

The Unspoken Message in Touch

Human beings communicate through touch on many different levels. A more casual form of touch might involve simply a handshake or a reassuring pat on the arm, whilst the manner in which we touch our partners, or children, might be more focused, and applied with more intention and care. Touch has the ability to communicate our feelings without words. Consider for a moment a parent crossing a busy road with a young child. As the adult quietly squeezes the child's hand more firmly, the parent is communicating their intention clearly through the medium of touch, and the child will often become aware of the message implied; *be safe and hang on tight!* What might the empathically driven reflexologist be communicating through their use of touch with a physically and emotionally exhausted client? What might the intention be? Perhaps to induce a similar sense of *'be safe, and hang on tight'*?

Summary

If I were being asked personally to define the concept of love within my reflexology practice my reply might be: *'I am present, I care, and my clients can feel that.'* Whilst it is unlikely concepts relating to love and conscious practitioner presence could be easily measured, or quantified, we can be fairly certain they represent a very real element impacting many reflexology exchanges. Understanding more about the limitations of love in reflexology certainly deserves more attention. The concept also clearly highlights the value of practitioner self development.

So is there a place for love in reflexology? I believe so, yes! Certainly, if *love* is to be defined as standing in a place of authentic concern for the unique individual, then it is perhaps simply a representation of our conscious presence and good intent within our professional boundaries. We must remain hopeful as our therapy strides forward in this modern world of clinical and scientific definitions that the transformative impact arising from authentic relating; where touch and pressure are utilised as a therapeutic medium, does not become too fleetingly acknowledged behind the mention of fibrous nerve tissue, fMRI scans, and autonomic system responses.

Reflexology is that, and much more. Reflexology is about connections, between the feet and body, *and* between two human beings. Love, care and intention impact both.

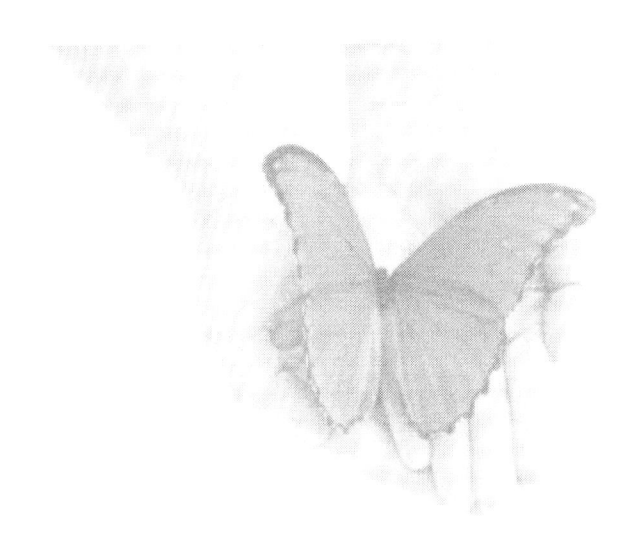

Relational Reflexology

The Multi-Dimensional Impact of Interpersonal Touch in Reflexology

"Touch has a memory."

- John Keats

Centrally positioned within the art of reflexology exists a well documented multi-dimensional concept connecting all forms of professional reflexology practice; that concept relates to interpersonal touch.

Researchers have extensively examined the importance of human interpersonal touch in mother/infant bonding, child development, and adult social interactions. The role of interpersonal touch as a counter-stimulation intervention in pain management (*Gate Control Theory*) has also been scientifically acknowledged. Additionally, the study of non-verbal communication is well established, with researchers possessing a high level of understanding concerning the subtle relationship between our inner emotions and desires, and that of our external posture, body language, and facial expressions. More recently researchers have been attempting to examine the innate human ability to non-verbally impart and decode emotional content through interpersonal touch.

"Human touch is a highly complex sensory modality, involving numerous interacting systems and exploratory capacities. Through touch we are able to interact with the world around us, feeling a wide variety of distinct properties, including warmth, solidity, roughness and elasticity. We use touch to conform and console each other, and touch is one of our primary conduits of pleasure and pain." (Fulkerson, 2014)

The intention of this chapter is to provide the reader with a glimpse into the scientific world of interpersonal touch. Touch as a therapeutic intervention is a much overlooked and entirely undervalued concept in modern reflexology, despite the provision of an extensive and wholly relevant body of work, open to reference. Developing a deeper understanding of the impact of interpersonal touch can certainly help reflexology practitioners to better understand the complexities and subtleties involved within our innately multi-dimensional modality, and to consider options for future reflexology research.

The Skin

The surface of the human body, the skin, is one enormous sheet of tactile receptors and constitutes by far the largest of our sense organs. The first sensations to develop in human beings are tactile, with researchers demonstrating a six week old foetus is able to react to tactile stimuli (Atkinson & Braddick, 1987; Bremmer et al., 2012)

"This complex system might be considered the most powerful interface ever designed between our self and the objects that surround us." (Gallace & Spence, 2014)

The skin provides us with a means of connecting with our external environment. It provides our body with protection, and it informs us about what is occurring on its surface (Gallace & Spence, 2014)

Tactile Receptors

Different tactile receptors innervate different parts of the skin. The level of sensitivity related to a particular region of the skin depends on the number of receptors within it.

Glabrous skin is only found on palms of the hands, soles of the feet, and parts of the genitals. Non glabrous skin (hairy skin) covers the rest of the body.

"It should be noted that the majority of studies of interpersonal touch have investigated the consequences of interpersonal touch on non-glabrous (hairy) skin sites." (Gallace & Spence, 2014)

Stimuli affecting both glabrous and hairy skin are translated into sensory neural signals by means of mechanoreceptors. Mechanoreceptors basically react to any mechanical stimulus delivered to the body surface (deformation of the skin). There are six classifications of tactile receptors:

- **Free Nerve Endings:** Found in hairy and glabrous skin. Sensitive to touch and pressure; situated in epidermal cells, and on the corneal surface of eye.

- **Root Hair Plexus:** Found in hairy skin. Monitors distortions and movements across the body surface.

- **Merkel Discs:** Found in glabrous skin. Sensitive to touch and pressure.

- **Meissner's Corpuscles:** Found in glabrous skin. Sensitive to fine touch, pressure and low frequency vibration.

- **Pacinian Corpuscles:** Found in hairy and glabrous skin. Sensitive to *deep pressure* and high frequency vibration (200-300hz); notably located in soles of feet, palms of hand, mammary glands, and external genitalia.

- **Ruffini Corpuscles:** Found in hairy and glabrous skin. Sensitive to pressure and distortion of the skin, located in the deep dermis.

Researchers classify mechanoreceptors as either *slow* or *rapidly* adapting. Both the **Pacinian** and the **Meissner** corpuscles (found in the feet and hands) are classified as *rapidly adapting*. This means these particular mechanoreceptors respond to the *onset* and *offset* of stimulation and cease discharging after a few seconds, rather than the slow adapting group of mechanoreceptors, which continue to respond for a certain amount of time under conditions of constant stimulation. (Gallace & Spence, 2014). This information perhaps highlights the possibility that the specific mechanical action associated with reflexology may be of particular importance. The thumb walking movement which define reflexology stimulation specifically seems to compliment the action of these particular mechanoreceptors. Additionally, researchers inform us the Pacinian corpuscles respond to deformation of the skin:

"such that the greater the deformation, the greater the generated potential." (Gallace & Spence, 2014)

Again, this perhaps hints towards suggesting the *depth* of pressure associated with reflexology may also be of particular significance.

Note: It is important to remember both glabrous and non-glabrous skin are located on the feet and hands, therefore reflexology is impacting all types of tactile receptor.

Touch and Psychoneuroimmunology

"People say the effect is only on the mind. It is no such thing. The effect is on the body, too." - Florence Nightingale

Psychoneuroimmunology (PNI) is an integrative scientific discipline. The research field seeks to explore how mental and emotional processes and events modulate the function of the immune system, and in turn how immunological activity can alter the function of the mind (Daruna, 2012). PNI postulates that persistent stress can increase the probability of developing many diseases, including cancer, coronary disease, and autoimmune disorders.

"The induction of relaxation, by any means, is associated with decreases in negative affect and counteracts sympathetic nervous system activity via the actions of nitric oxide. Relaxation also produces alterations of hormone levels in the circulation. Consequently, effects on immune activity would be expected." (Daruna, 2012)

The effects of tactile contact have been documented in a variety of health-care related behaviours. For example, researchers (Whitcher & Fisher, 1979; Wong, Ghiasuddin, Kimata, Patelesio, & Siu, 2013), demonstrated the act of receiving touch from a nurse the day prior to surgery can result in a decrease in the patients stress levels when measured both objectively (heart rate/blood pressure), and subjectively (patient evaluation).

Interpersonal touch has been clinically proven to aid the release of endorphins, in addition to the neuropeptides, serotonin, and dopamine. When released into the bloodstream these chemicals serve to counteract and suppress the effects of adrenal stress hormones, cortisol and adrenaline (Field, Hernandez-Reif, & Diego, 2005).

"The tactile information processing system is likely more closely linked to the neural systems that support hormonal responses than to any other sensory system in the brain." (Gallace & Spence).

Research also suggests interpersonal touch induces oxytocin release in humans. Oxytocin is produced by the hypothalamus, and transported to, and secreted by the posterior adrenal gland. Both a hormone and a neurotransmitter, oxytocin has been proven to reduce stress response and feelings of anxiety (Newman, 2007, Churchland, 2011). Oxytocin is perhaps most associated with the neuroanatomy of intimacy, specifically sexual reproduction, facilitating childbirth, maternal bonding, and, after stimulation of the nipples, lactation.

Scientific research is also beginning to discover more about oxytocin's role in modulating social behaviour, including maternal bonding, couples bonding, sexual behaviour, social memory, and even trust (Newman, 2007). A number of studies have investigated the role of touch between intimate partners in mediating the release of oxytocin (Bales & Carter, 2003; Bielsky & Young, 2004; Carter, 1998, 1999; Cho, De Vries, Williams, & Carter, 1999; Feldman, 2012). Holt-Lunstad et al, (2008), for example, found that couples who engaged in an exercise involving touching each other's necks, shoulders, and hands, displayed higher levels of oxytocin in their saliva than couples who did not engage in the touch exercise. Another study (Light et al, 2005), demonstrated that women who report frequent partner hugs display higher levels of oxytocin in their blood than women who report fewer partner hugs. Researchers believe the release of oxytocin can help couples to form lasting relationship bonds (Gulledge et al., 2007).

Touch and Pain Responses

"Now while we know the fact of pain relief, through the laying on of hands, or by kindred measures, we know only a part of its reason for operation. There are several of these. They are, first, the soothing influence of animal magnetism, experienced when we tenderly, if not lovingly, rub the bump, accumulated in the dark of the moon, by a collision with a tall brunette side-board, or a door carelessly left ajar. It does soothe. This we know." - William Fitzgerald (1919)

The Gate Control Theory of Pain was introduced in the 1960s by Ronald Melzack and Patrick Wall. The theory identifies the experience of pain as a complex interplay between the central and peripheral nervous systems. When physical injury occurs, messages travel along the peripheral nerves to the spinal cord, and then on to the brain.

Before pain messages are able to reach the brain they encounter nerve 'gates' (*inhibitory neural mechanisms*) located in the spinal cord. When the nerve gates are open pain messages rapidly reach the brain, and when the gates are closed messages are hindered in reaching their destination.

"Stress causes changes in the activity of the autonomic nervous system (ANS) and, more generally, the peripheral nervous system (PNS)." (Daruna, 2012)

The underlying principle in Gate Control Theory is to introduce factors capable of closing the pain gates. These factors might be physiologically or psychologically based and can include focused concentration, relaxation, distraction, mediation, exercise, and tactile counter-stimulation (reflexology, massage, TENS etc).

There are two types of nerve fibres carrying the majority of pain messages to the spinal cord:

- **A-delta** Fibers - carry electrical messages to the spinal cord at approximately 40 mph.

- **C-Fibers** - carry electrical messages to the spinal cord at approximately 3 mph.

"The delivery of a single painful stimulus will evoke two successive and qualitatively distinct sensations referred to as first and second pain. First pain is brief, pricking, and well localised on the skin surface, and its perception results from the activation of myelinated A-delta fibers. Second pain is longer-lasting, burning, associated with a burning sensation, and tends to be less well localised. It results from activation of unmyelinated C-fibers that conduct the neural signal more slowly than the A-fibers." (Gallace & Spence, 2014).

William Fitzgerald's loving rub after his bump into the tall brunette side-board provides us with a good example of how these respective nerve fibres operate. The initial bump causes activation of the A-delta nerve fibers. Fitzgerald instinctively follows the event with a 'rub' of the area, thus activating even faster nerve fibers to send information spinal cord and brain, in turn overriding some of the pain messages carried by the A-delta and C-fibers (closing their passage to the central nervous system). And so it soothes!

Carol Samuel, a UK reflexology researcher, recently carried out a small study (Samuel & Ebenezer, 2013) examining the effects of reflexology on acute pain responses. Dr Samuel asked volunteer participants to place their hands into ice cold water and two measurements of pain were noted: threshold (first indications of pain) and tolerance (the time at which the participants could no longer tolerate any further pain). Findings concluded:

"Reflexology produces antinociceptive effects in a controlled experiment and suggest the possibility that reflexology may be useful on its own or as an adjunct to medication in the treatment of pain conditions in man."

In another small study (Stephenson, 2003) cancer patients were offered reflexology twice in 24 hours. This study demonstrated:

"immediate positive effect of reflexology for patients with metatstatic cancer who report pain."

Note: 'Antinociceptive' describes or relates to any unique factor that increases tolerance for, or reduces sensitivity to, a dangerous or harmful stimuli, for example, a stimuli that may cause pain.

Touch and Child Development

"The evidence indicates that grooming maintains social relationships between nonhuman primates of every age, sex, and rank. It is plausible that humans' tactile communication system may have evolved from the intricate system of tactile content evident in nonhuman primates." (Hertenstein et al. 2009)

One of the most famous (and possibly cruel) touch related studies was carried out during the 1950s by the American psychologist Harry Harlow. The study was designed to examine how touch might influence infant coping mechanisms. Harlow raised baby Rhesus monkeys in a cage housing two surrogate 'mothers'; one surrogate constructed from metal wire held a feeding bottle while the other surrogate was wrapped in terrycloth. As the baby monkeys became frightened they clung to the terrycloth surrogate, even though that meant they became dehydrated and starved. Harlow used these studies to demonstrate that intimate body contact, and not feeding, was the most important factor in mother-child bonding.

John Bowlby (1973) is the British psychiatrist responsible for the psychological/developmental concept called attachment theory. Attachment theory suggests that touch provided by primary care givers enables infants to feel safe and secure, and thus provides the foundation for all securely attached relationships formed in later life. Many subsequent studies have gone on to confirm Bowlby's pioneering work.

"Touch is central to human social life. It is the most developed sensory modality at birth, and it contributes to cognitive, brain, and socioemotional development throughout infancy and childhood." (Hertenstein et al. 2006)

One study (DeAngelis & Mwakalyelye, 1995) concluded babies stroked regularly were healthier and thrived better than those babies receiving no touch. This study interestingly additionally concluded those mothers who received massage were less depressed and anxious than those receiving relaxation training only.

Similarly, a study carried out by Wiess et al. (2000) found that a mothers nurturing touch was able to foster more secure attachment in low birth weight infants, nine months later. An Australian study, (Paslow, Morgan, Allan, Jorm, O'Donnell, & Purcell, 2007), reviewing the effectiveness of complementary therapies for anxiety in both children and adolescents demonstrated massage had immediate and short-term effects on anxiety.

Touch into Adulthood

Researchers believe the soothing effects of interpersonal touch remain important throughout adulthood, both in a social interaction context, and within the context of interpersonal relationships. Many social psychology studies have highlighted the manner in which interpersonal touch can help to regulate social interactions and relationships. Researchers have identified that touch can even influence the social behaviours of a person, inducing them to sign a petition (Willis & Hamm, 1980), return lost money (Kleinke, 1977), leave a bigger tip (Crusco & Wetzel, 1984), and, motivate people to work harder on shared tasks (Gueguen, 2004).

Another interesting study (Eaton, Mitchell-Bonair, & Friedmann) demonstrated that when staff in a care home touched elderly patients at the same time as verbally encouraging them to eat, the patients consumed more calories and protein for five days after the touch. A study by (Grewen, Anderson, Girdler, Light, 2003) revealed individuals who received pre-stress tactile partner contact demonstrated significantly lower systolic and diastolic blood pressure and heart rate increases than the no contact group.

Similarly, Ditzen et al. (2007) investigated whether specific kinds of physical interaction between couples can reduce hypothalamic-pituitary-adrenal (HPA) and autonomic responses to psychosocial stress in women. The participants were randomly assigned to one of three control groups: no interaction with their partner, verbal interaction with their partner, physical contact with their partner, before being exposed to a stressor event.

The results revealed those women experiencing physical contact demonstrated significantly lower cortisol and heart rate responses to the stressor event.

Communicating Emotion via Interpersonal Touch

More recently researchers have been trying to understand the complex relationship between interpersonal touch and human emotions. One fascinating study (Hertenstein et al, 2006) required pairs of participants to be seated at a table separated by a curtain, and unable to see each other. One participant (the encoder) was asked to communicate distinct emotions by touching the other participants forearm. The person being touched (the decoder) was asked to try and identify the communicated emotion from a number of offered response options.

The results suggest human beings come readily equipped with an innate ability to send and receive emotional signals through touch. In fact, participants in this study were able to communicate eight distinct emotions: anger, fear, disgust, love, gratitude, sympathy, happiness, and sadness. The research team expected accuracy rates to display at around chance level (25%), but were in fact as high as 78%. Such remarkable findings allowed the team to suggest interpersonal touch is important to emotional communication, and potentially intimately involved in the expression of positive emotions between people.

A team from the same research facility latterly carried out a similar study (Hertenstein et al. 2009). In this experiment participants were required to touch an unacquainted partner on the body to communicate emotion. The encoder entered the room to find the decoder standing blindfolded. The encoder was randomly shown one of eight emotions on a piece of paper and asked to think about how they wanted to communicate the chosen emotion, before touching the decoder on an appropriate part of the body.

This study concluded that touch communicates eight emotions: anger, fear, happiness, sadness, disgust, love, gratitude, and sympathy. Accuracy rates in this study ranged on average from 50-70%. Researchers additionally concluded that touch demonstrates greater differentiation (of emotion) than the voice, and perhaps the face.

"Emotional/hedonistic touch can be differentiated from perceptual touch at many different levels of neural processing." (Gallace & Spence, 2014)

Another study (Gazzola, et al., 2012) used fMRI to measure brain activity in individuals receiving interpersonal touch. The participants, all heterosexual males, were shown a video of a man or a woman appearing to touch their leg. The videos however were faked and the real touch was provided by a woman who remained shielded from the study participant's view.

Study findings revealed the participants, perhaps unsurprisingly, rated the experience of male touch as less pleasant than that of the female touch. Perhaps more interestingly, the fMRI scans highlighted that part of the brain called the primary somatosensory cortex showed increased activity when the participants received what they *perceived* as female touch.

These findings are particularly important because prior to this study researchers believed the primary somatosensory cortex was responsible for encoding only very basic qualities of touch, such as pressure, or texture, however, because brain activity was being influenced by the participants *perception* of who they thought was touching them the study was able to conclude that emotional and social components of touch are absolutely related to tactile sensation, and thus the experience of touch is affected by the individuals *social evaluation* of the person providing the touch.

Therapeutic Touch (TT)

Therapeutic Touch was pioneered by Delores Kreiger, a Professor of Nursing at New York University, and is widely integrating into nursing in the USA and Canada. Therapeutic touch can be distinguished from most other bio-energetic therapies because the modality has been demonstrated to be effective after extensive, empirical investigation (Graham, 1999). Therapeutic Touch can be carried out using physical or non-physical contact. In essence the practitioner is attempting to focus their attention towards achieving a relaxed and focused state in which they make an assessment of the patient's energetic body field. The practitioner attempts to achieve this stance through developing an awareness of *sensations* in their own hands and body. The patients affected area is balanced using colour imagery as a focus for directing healing energies, for example, red to warm and stimulate an area, blue to cool or sedate, yellow to energise. When the practitioner becomes aware of the patients energetic body field starting to feel more balanced, the healing session is considered complete.

A 2009 study reviewing prior research relating to the effects of therapeutic touch on pain recommended grounds for implementing TT as a pain management intervention because of:

"a majority of statistically significant positive results' (Monroe, 2009)

Note: Whilst Therapeutic Touch differs from reflexology in that it offers no direct stimulation to the tissues of the body, it does share certainly a similar focus of intention stemming from the practitioner. The concept of transferring emotional or energetic content between client and practitioner can also be found within a counselling and psychotherapy context (i.e. transference/counter-transference).

Summary

"The science of touch convincingly suggests that we're wired to - we need to - connect with other people on a basic physical level. To deny that is to deprive ourselves of some of life's greatest joys and deepest comforts." - Dacher Keltner

In medieval Europe rich nobles were reported to have slept in beds large enough to accommodate their wife, children, servants, and even their knights. This close proximity sleeping arrangement offered a perfect protection against the icy chills of winter. Across the centuries, influenced by the fluctuating nature of social and cultural norms, many forms of interpersonal touch have become less common. Indeed, the idea of sleeping on mass today might be considered as unhygienic, invasive and inappropriate. Sadly, gone too are the days where the empathetic nursery nurse or teacher might freely offer a kindly hug to an emotionally distressed child. Human beings seem to be more isolated within their own personal space, and detached from instinctual acts of interpersonal touch than at any other time in history. Perhaps this trend towards social and physical isolation provides a rationale for why human beings are so drawn towards healing modalities such as reflexology? Being touched it would seem is an innate requirement for many human beings, from the cradle to the grave.

There are many complementary modalities offering interpersonal touch to clients, however, reflexology undoubtedly stands alone in its capacity to offer a combination of interpersonal touch, focused intention, and the benefit of an emotionally supportive therapeutic relationship. Reflexology impacts both body and mind in a complex, multi-dimensional manner. The scientific principles of psychoneuroimmunology, and the close working relationship between the psychological, immunological, and cognitive neuroscience communities, are helping to highlight the underlying principles of many holistic mind/body modalities.

- Reflexologists **touch:** research is helping us to understand how that touch is impacting our clients neurological, endocrine, and psychological processes.

- Reflexologists work with **intention:** new research is helping us to better understand how that intention within our touch can be decoded by the receiver.

- Reflexologists **listen**, **empathise** and even **educate:** research is helping us to understand more about how stress and emotional states can impact physiology, and about how supportive therapeutic relationships can help to promote autonomy and self-directed change.

"No single science approaches completeness. A little knowledge here and a little there applied to whatever method you may already be using to help suffering humanity may prove a priceless asset to your success." - Eunice D. Ingham

No single field of research relies solely upon its own findings, nor should reflexology. There is an enormous difference between personal opinion, and factual verified information. As the modality moves forward in attempting to refine the definition of reflexology we should endeavour to embrace the findings of the wider scientific community. There seems to be a concern present within parts of our industry that in embracing scientific or academic information we may be in danger of losing, or become detached from, the metaphysical core principles of the modality. On the contrary, as is blindingly transparent from the information presented, the scientific research community is undoubtedly only better informing our intellectual understanding of reflexology.

The language used may differ somewhat. The reflexologist might refer to intention or energy transfer, whilst the cognitive neuroscientist or psychologist might refer to encoded and decoded information. Perhaps though in truth the only difference is in the language?

Certainly, for the time-being at least, neither group can claim to truly understand the origins of such energy/information, but we are certainly becoming clearer about its potential impact. As professional reflexologists we should embrace scientific research, embrace knowledge, and in doing so embrace a renewed understanding of the multi-dimensional impact of the reflexology package.

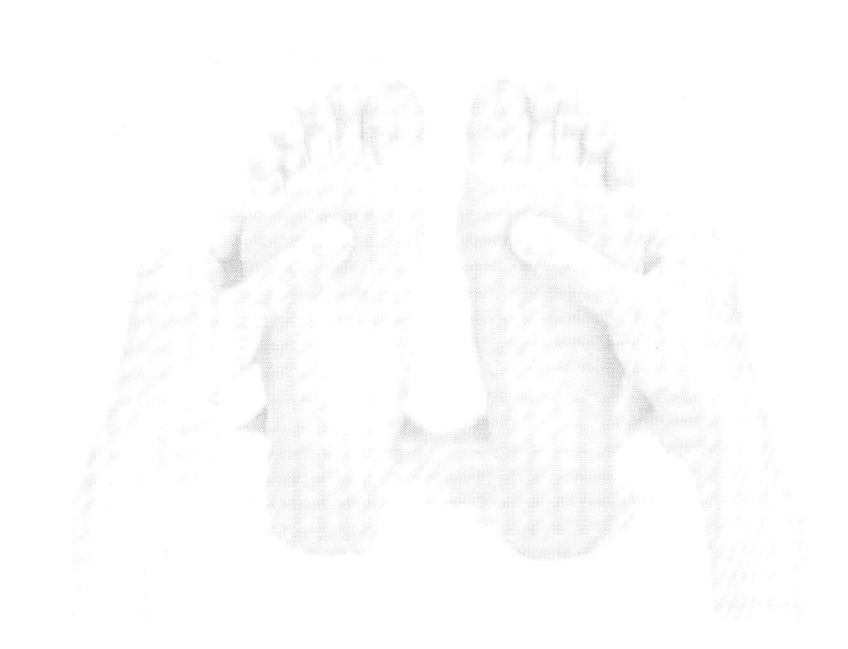

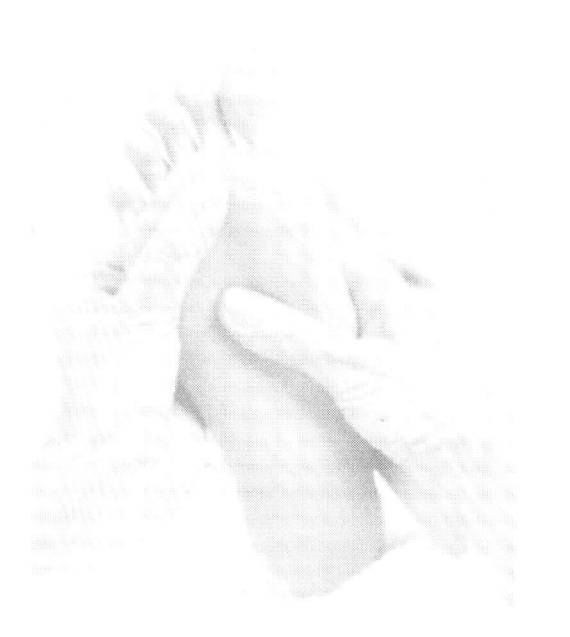

Relational Reflexology

Wired for Compassion – The Human Brain and the Supportive Reflexology Package

*"Love and compassion are necessities, not luxuries.
Without them, humanity cannot survive."*

- Dalai Lama

At first glance compassion might appear a difficult to measure, rather subjective subject, however, the concept has certainly attracted a great deal of research attention across recent years, principally because of the close philosophical association between compassionate states, and the Buddhist practice of mindfulness. The intention of this article is to explore the manner in which the human brain and nervous system responds to witnessing suffering in others, and to highlight the positive role of compassion in human health.

Additionally, the intention is to offer the reader an opportunity to consider how their own feelings of compassion might impact reflexology clients, and finally, to champion the reflexology package as a powerful multi-dimensional therapeutic balm; capable of soothing individual instances of personal suffering through tactile interpersonal touch, and the practitioners engagement in active states of compassion and empathy.

Compassion and the Theory of Human Evolution

Many people tend to associate Charles Darwin with the somewhat dominant phrase; *'survival of the fittest'*. You might be surprised to learn however these are not in fact Darwin's words. The phrase was actually coined by later Darwinists in attempts to justify their own particular views on social and race issues of the time. In fact, rather than supporting the notion of survival of the fittest, Darwin conversely theorised those communities comprising of more sympathetic individuals tended to be more successful in raising healthy offspring to a viable age of reproduction. To help form his opinions, Darwin drew not only upon observations of his own children, but also observations of animals at London zoo, and even his own pet dogs, before concluding all mammals feel some degree of sympathy, and, that mammalian expressions of sympathy tend to be played out through social forms of tactile contact (social grooming/interpersonal touch).

"We have seen that the senses and intuitions, the various emotions and faculties, such as love, memory, attention and curiosity, imitation, reason, etc., of which man boasts, may be found in an incipient, or even sometimes in a well-developed condition, in the lower animals." - Charles Darwin

As our ancestors began to walk upright, and the human brain grew in size, so too the human pelvis narrowed. These enormous evolutionary changes prompted the necessity for human babies to be birthed at an earlier stage in their cognitive development, enabling the large human head to pass safely through the narrow birth canal. The human infant is born entirely vulnerable and dependant on adult care givers and compassionate instincts, whilst conversely, baby chimpanzees are able to feed independently at a much earlier age, and can sit unsupported without fear of toppling over.

To accommodate for the increased levels of care required by human offspring, more complex care-taking social structures began to emerge, and perhaps unsurprisingly, evolution also enhanced the human nervous system to ensure the presence of appropriate care-taking responses.

Compassion and the Brain

"Consider these empirical findings: When people perform altruistic acts, the same regions of their brain light up as when they receive rewards or experience pleasure; humans are equipped with specialised "mirror neurons" that enable us to empathise with others; we produce the hormone oxytocin, which promotes social bonding, trust, and

generosity; and activation of our vagus nerve, a bundle of nerves near the spinal cord, increases compassion and cooperation." - Dacher Keltner

With the help of modern neuroscience researchers are beginning to understand in more depth the manner in which the human brain responds to the experience of witnessing suffering in others. Studies have discovered when an individual reacts to physical pain activity is noted in a part of the brain called the *anterior cingulate*. Researchers have also discovered this part of the brain not only reacts to our own personal pain, but also as we witness pain in others.

Scientists refer to some of the neurons firing in this part of the brain as *mirror neurons*. Researchers believe because these neurons fire when witnessing another's pain or suffering they may somehow be involved in the experience of *empathy*, as well as mimicking, goal achieving, and understanding an action.

The *amygdala* also reacts to suffering in others. The amygdala is described as the part of the brain's threat/fear detector. Researchers believe because this part of the brain helps us to identify possible threats, it also therefore alerts us to the possibility that we may be about to experience suffering.

Finally, another very old part of the mammalian nervous system called the *periaqueductal gray*, an anatomic and functional interface between the forebrain and the lower brainstem also shows activity when suffering is witnessed in others. This area of the brain plays a role in the descending modulation of pain, defensive behaviour and in the mammal kingdom is also associated with nurturing.

Compassion and the Vagus Nerve

This vagus nerve (or 10th cranial nerve) has been dubbed one of the great mind-body nexuses in the human body. The vagus nerve is a mixed nerve, with both sensory and motor functions. It is the longest of the cranial nerves extending from the brain stem, to the muscles of the mouth, neck, thorax, lungs, and abdomen. Branches of the vagus nerve extend to:

- Auricular nerve
- Pharyngeal nerve
- Superior laryngeal nerve
- Superior cervical cardiac branches of the vagus nerve
- Inferior cervical cardiac branch
- Recurrent laryngeal nerve
- Thoracic cardiac branches
- Branches to the pulmonary plexus
- Branches to the esophageal plexus
- Anterior vagal trunk
- Posterior vagal trunk
- Hering breuer reflex in alveoli

The vagus nerve is associated with:

- Regulating muscles in the neck responsible for nodding the head, orienting the gaze, voice resonance, and the soft palate.
- Coordinating interactions of the cardiovascular system.
- Homeostasis of the digestive tract, the stomach, spleen, liver, and lower digestive processes.
- Oxytocin release.
- Immune system response.
- Inflammation response.

In essence the vagus nerve responds to our conscious awareness of the environment around us. Depending on the brains assessment of the environment, the vagus nerve either responds by supporting homeostasis in the associated systems and organs, or the nervee can react to stressor events by elevating all associated autonomic responses.

"To perceive is to suffer." — Aristotle

In addition to reacting to our own personal evaluations, researchers have also discovered when study participants are shown photographs or videos of suffering and distress, or are told a sad, or even inspiring story, their vagus nerve responds. Indeed, scientists now believe the stronger the feelings of compassion in the individual, the more intense the vagus nerve response.

It would appear human beings have indeed been evolutionary hard-wired to recognise and respond to the suffering of our fellow man.

Compassion and Empathy

The term empathy is generally defined as the ability to sense another persons emotions, coupled with the ability to imagine what someone else might be thinking or feeling. Contemporary emotion researchers tend to differentiate between two types of empathy:

Affective empathy: refers to the sensations and feelings brought about in the self in response to experiencing others' emotion. This can include physically and/or emotionally experiencing what the other person is feeling.

Cognitive empathy: refers to the ability to interpret, identify, and intellectually understand others' experience and emotions. This is sometimes also referred to as perspective taking.

Within a reflexology context it is possible both forms of empathy are present in varying degrees. Affective empathy with its associated bodily sensations and physiological impact can be defined as experienced in both the visceral and emotional dimensions (perhaps defined alternatively by many reflexology practitioners as an energy rush/transfer).

The presence of cognitive empathy tends to develop as a result of practitioner/client verbal interactions, and client emotional disclosure.

Empathy and the Therapeutic Relationship

"Too often we underestimate the power of a touch, a smile, a kind word, a listening ear, an honest compliment, or the smallest act of caring, all of which have the potential to turn a life around." - Leo Buscaglia

Carl Rogers (1951), the founder of *Person Centred Therapy* believed unconditional positive regard, congruence and empathy to be the qualities required to form effective therapeutic relationships. These core therapeutic conditions are often referred to as ways of being. Ideally the practitioner is striving to provide a safe space in which the client experiences unconditional warmth, and acceptance. No demands, or expectations are placed upon the client and they are free to be their real authentic self, and are valued as such. The practitioner attempts to demonstrate their empathic understanding of the client's unique frame of reference, mindful, that for every individual the experience of life (and health) is entirely unique, regardless the commonality of experience.

Empathy essentially begins from a place of **awareness**. Sometimes our awareness develops through asking clarifying questions, sometimes we use our intuition and read between the lines, and sometimes we might interpret more non-verbal, physical clues. On some occasions we might encounter very emotionally expressive people; those who seem able to tell a fuller story through their facial expressions and eyes.

To empathise is also to **acknowledge** our awareness. For example, a client might describe how frustrated they feel about an enforced change of position at work, and the practitioner might choose to reflect their own empathic understanding of that expressed frustration.

Practitioner: *"I can appreciate how difficult you are finding the changes."*

Whilst telling their story the client might become agitated, angry, or perhaps even weepy, or deflated. To acknowledge the presence of an emotion or a sense of exhaustion is also to empathise.

Practitioner: *"I can see from your posture how agitated/deflated the situation seems to have left you feeling."*

Practitioner: *"I can hear in your tone of voice how agitated/deflated the situation seems to have left you feeling."*

Compassion and the Mind

There is an unfortunate trend in reflexology towards considering clients as defined by a clinical diagnosis, or reported condition. This stance of practice unfortunately often dictates the application of reflexology becomes a procedure; defined as a series of specific reflex points to be stimulated prescriptively. This form of practice clearly lacks any real empathic connection with the client. Dealing with client emotional content in reflexology can present a similar challenge. How can practitioners remain connected to the client's unique experience, and not assume the place of an authority figure?

Many reflexology practitioners quite understandably wish to develop their therapist tool box to include an awareness of how to safely use basic psychological interventions. The theoretical core principles contextualised as the therapeutic relationship certainly offer professional practitioners a safe means of developing more meaningful, empathically driven, interpersonal connections. Clients receiving this type of approach are also often more likely to engage in the co-operative healing process, prompted by feeling supported, involved, and active within the therapeutic relationship.

It is possible one of the main benefits of the reflexology package might the rapid focus of attention brought to the client's physical body responses (the felt sense). The inclusion therefore of any additional intervention capable of further promoting reconnection of the mind-body (psycho-soma) state (i.e. mindfulness activities/focused breathing/steeping the feet/tapping), can certainly *complement* the action of reflexology. On the other hand, some of the more directive psychological interventions, particularly those where focus is placed upon inner narrative and rational decision making (i.e. CBT type interventions) may well prove to be *counter-productive* to the action of reflexology (due to the singular focus of attention placed on cognitive processes), and should therefore be avoided.

A great deal of counselling and psychotherapy research suggests the most important factor in a successful therapy encounter is not the model of counselling or psychotherapy utilised, but rather the *quality* of the therapeutic relationship. **Empathy** and **compassion** are pillars of the therapeutic relationship. Within a good quality therapeutic relationship the client remains the expert in their own life and experiencing (promoting an active, rather than passive stance), and the practitioners role is to listen, empathise, and touch; perhaps just as nature intended.

Emotion in Touch

"There is increasing evidence for a different central neural representation to stroking either glabrous or hairy skin, in normal populations, in limbic rather than primary somatosensory structure." (McGlone, et all, 2007)

Researchers studying the affective aspects of tactile content suggest the brains *insular cortex* may play an important role in processing our emotional, hormonal, and affiliative responses to touch (Gallace and Spence, 2014). The insular cortex is believed to be involved in consciousness, and plays a role in diverse functions linked to emotion, and the regulation of homeostasis in the body. This part of the brain is believed to process signals arising from different sensory channels, and thus also helps to co-ordinate an appropriate emotional response to any given sensory experience.

"Our brains appear to discriminate between interpersonal touch, interpersonal touch, and the passive touch of an object or surface on the skin." (Gallace & Spence, 2014)

Gazzola et al., (2012), used fMRI scans to measure brain activity in individuals receiving interpersonal touch. This study was able to conclude that emotional and social components of touch are absolutely intwined with tactile sensations, and thus the experience of touch is affected by the individual's social evaluation of the person providing the touch (*for details see interpersonal touch chapter*).

"The meaning of touch is something that goes far beyond the stimulation of the skins surface and this is why our experience of it is affected by our beliefs, or expectations (be they right or wrong), regarding who it is who is doing the touching, and why." – Gallace & Spence (2014)

Only a few cognitive neuroscience studies have investigated whether skin to skin contact is processed by the brain in a different manner to touch applied by means of an inanimate object. One study (Kress et al., 2012) examined how the brain interpreted touch when delivered by the experimenter's hand, compared to touch delivered by a velvet covered stick.

The fMRI results from this study demonstrated that touch applied with the human hand elicited larger responses in the primary and secondary somatosensory areas of the brain. The research team suggested this effect was at least partially mediated by the participant's cognitive and emotional *perception* of human interpersonal touch. Findings seem to suggest the *primary somatosensory cortex* is responsible for initially registering the physiological mechanics of touch, before the impulse is transmitted to other parts of the brain, where the more affiliative aspects of touch seem to be processed.

Research carried out in the field of social psychology (Hertenstein et al., 2006 & Hertenstein et al., 2009) demonstrated that human beings possess an innate ability to impart and decode emotional content from fairly brief instances of interpersonal touch, at well above chance levels (*for details see interpersonal touch chapter*).

Summary

Many practitioners associated with mind/body modalities may have acknowledged for example, the impact of emotional distress on the function of the human digestive system. Certainly a large percentage of practitioners will have encountered the reflexology client so anxious in their disposition they complain of daily acid knots in the stomach, or the IBS client who reports distress regarding their child's impending departure to university, or perhaps a change of role at work. New information explaining the function of structures such as the vagus nerve appears to be providing an element of scientific validation to many long held holistic beliefs.

The ancient prophecy of the Eagle and the Condor tells of human societies splitting to follow two very different paths. The path of the Condor is associated with the human heart, compassion, intuition, and the feminine. The path of the Eagle is associated with the human mind, logic, the physical world, and the masculine. The prophecy states after a 500 year separation (beginning around 1490) the potential would arise once again for the Eagle and the Condor to come together in the same sky, and in doing so, create a new level of consciousness for humanity.

"Until he extends the circle of his compassion to all living things, man will not himself find peace." – Albert Schweitzer

The complex human brain has evolved to respond positively to the most subjective of therapeutic interventions; sympathy, compassion, and care. In mammalian species acts of demonstrative compassion tend to involve tactile content (social grooming/interpersonal touch); certainly a more measurable concept.

In summary, the reflexology package seems perfectly constructed to provide both tactile physical stimulation, and the human qualities of compassion, empathy, and care. Responses often craved during times of emotional distress. Scientific validation of the mind-body connection is undoubtedly still in its infancy, but the concept is certainly alive and well within research communities. With exciting developments in cognitive neuroscience, and the merging of previously fragmented scientific disciplines (psychoneuroimmunology), perhaps it really is time for the Eagle and the Condor to share the sky once again?

The future certainly looks bright for reflexology.

Relational Reflexology

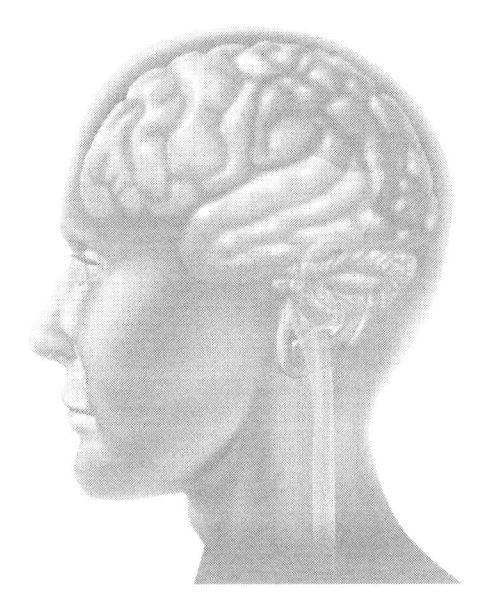

The Brain, Electrical Impulses, Chemical Communications and Reflexology

"The root of all health is in the brain. The trunk of it is in emotion. The branches and leaves are the body. The flower of health blooms when all parts work together."

- Kurdish Saying

The brain is the most sophisticated entity known to man. The human brain measures approximately the size and shape of a cauliflower, and weighs around 1.36kg (3lb). Although the brain makes up only 2% of human body weight it consumes 20% of the average human's daily energy intake.

Scientists first began attempting to map the territory of the brain in the 19th century. Initially, information was gathered through animal experiments, and by examining the brains of deceased individuals with some form of brain damage. It has only become possible over the last 25 years for scientists to more fully investigate the brain structure and function in healthy volunteers.

Architecture of the Brain

The Forebrain

The forebrain is known as **prosencephalon**. It is responsible for a variety of functions including receiving and processing sensory information, thinking, perceiving, producing and understanding language, and controlling motor function. There are two major divisions of forebrain:

- The **diencephalon** contains the thalamus and hypothalamus, responsible for motor control, relaying sensory information, and controlling autonomic function.

- The **telencephalon** contains the cerebrum. Much of the information processing in the brain takes place within the cerebral cortex.

The Cerebral Cortex

The cerebral cortex refers to the deeply folded outer layers of the brain. It accounts for two thirds of brain volume and houses the majority of the grey matter in the brain. The cerebral cortex is divided into two hemispheres, and again further into lobes.

Frontal Lobes - The most highly developed in humans compared with other animal species. The two frontal lobes are associated with **decision making, memory, planning, voluntary action**, and **personality.**

Occipital Lobes - Located at the back of the brain the two occipital lobes are mainly involved in **vision**.

Parietal Lobes - Located above the occipital lobes and behind the frontal lobes (crown of the head). The parietal lobes are deeply involved in integrating **sensory information**.

Temporal Lobes - Located low to the side of each hemisphere (near the ears), the temporal lobes are involved in **object recognition, memory formation, storage,** and **language.**

Situated within the many folds of the cerebral cortex are other mapped and named areas of the brain. Each respective area is further associated with more specific actions and systems.

The Thalamus

The thalamus is a bundle of neurons (nuclei) located at the top of the brain stem. The thalamus nuclei are heavily interconnected with specific areas of the cerebral cortex, and are believed to act as sensory relay areas, connecting sensory receptors (apart from olfaction) within the cortex.

The Hypothalamus

The hypothalamus plays a major role in regulating hormones, the pituitary gland, body temperature, the adrenal glands, and many other vital activities. The hypothalamus is also an important emotional centre, responsible for controlling molecules associated with feelings of exhilaration, anger, or sadness.

The Midbrain

The midbrain is known as the **mesencephalon** and is located near the centre of the brain between the interbrain and the hindbrain, and comprises a portion of the brainstem. This region of the brain is associated with auditory and visual sensory responses, and motor function.

The Hindbrain

The hindbrain is known as the **rhombencephalon** and consists of two parts:

1. A sub-region of the hindbrain referred to as **myelencephalon**.

The Brain Stem

The brain stem is a small stalk like area located between the bottom of the brain and the **spinal cord**. It is divided across three structures the midbrain, pons, and medulla oblongata. The brainstem houses many of the control centres for vital body functions, such as swallowing, breathing, and vasomotor control.

All of the cranial nerve nuclei, with the exception of those associated with olfaction and vision are located in the brainstem.

The Medulla Oblongata

The medulla oblongata is responsible for controlling autonomic functions such as breathing, heart rate, and digestion.

2. A second area of the hindbrain housing the cerebellum and pons is referred to as the **metencephalon**.

The Cerebellum

The cerebellum is often referred to as the 'little brain'. The cerebellum accounts for 10% of the brain's volume, yet contains around half the neurons found in the entire central nervous system. The cerebellum is also constructed of two hemispheres, and joined by a narrow structure called the vermis. The cerebellum cortex is made up of while matter in its deeper parts and grey matter near to its surface. This part of the brain is primarily associated with motor control, co-ordination and the formation of forward models of prediction. The cerebellum is also becoming increasingly associated with memory, mood, language, and attention.

The Pons

The pons, or pons varolii, is a part of the brainstem linking the medulla oblongata with the thalamus.

Other Important Structures

The Insular Cortex

"Studies suggest that C fibers have a primary cortical target in the posterior insular cortex. That is the system responsible for pleasant touch is activated by the stimulation of C-fibers is likely to be a complex network associated with the maintenance of physical and social well-being in humans." (Gallace & Spence, 2014)

The insular cortex (or insula) is a potion of the cerebral cortex folded deep within the lateral sulcus, at the bottom of the junction of the temporal, parietal, and frontal lobes. The insular cortex is involved in detecting and representing the internal state of the body (interoception).

The insular cortex is believed to contribute to the processing of signals arising from different sensory channels to produce an emotionally relevant response, and so is associated with conscious emotional experience and self awareness. Other functions include motor control and cognitive functioning.

Researchers studying the neural correlates of the more affective aspects of touch suggest the insular cortex to be an important system responsible for our emotional, hormonal, and affiliative responses to tactile behaviours related to social grooming and nurture.

"One might therefore hypothesise that part of the neural network responsible for the processing of certain emotional aspects of tactile experiences is actually shared with the network responsible for processing information from other sensory modalities." (Gallace and Spence, 2014)

Only a few studies have utilised fMRI to assess whether the emotional aspect of skin to skin touch is processed in a different manner to that provided by an inanimate object. For example, Kress, Minati, Ferraro, and Critchley (2012) found stroking with the hand elicited a larger response in the contralateral primary, and secondary somatosensory areas, as well as the posterior insula.

Alberto Gallace (2014), a neuroscientist and expert in the field of interpersonal touch research offered during email communication with the writer, his conviction that:

"The same signal from the peripheral receptors can be interpreted very differently as a function of the context. And the social context is probably the most effective in modulating the interpretation and the consequences of the signals."

This information presents us with two interesting concepts to reflect upon. The first is to acknowledge the brain's interpretation of touch is dependent on the individual's social perception of the person providing the touch. The second is to consider how to factor this into our intellectual interpretation of reflexology and how to further represent this within reflexology research.

Alberto Gallace believes because the affiliative responses to touch develop earlier in human beings it:

"is probably more powerful than perceptual touch"

Consider, a new born infant will develops their awareness of interpersonal touch much sooner than an awareness of perceptual touch. Humans require caring affiliative touch long before their requirement to stand, walk, balance, and judge their environment.

The Cingulate Cortex

The cingulate cortex is located in the medial aspect of the cerebral cortex, and considered an integral part of the *limbic system*. The cingulate cortex is comprised of two parts: posterior (back) and anterior (front).

The anterior cingulate cortex is linked to several autonomic functions, such as regulating blood pressure and heart rate, anticipation, decision-making and emotional responses. Imaging studies indicate the posterior cingulate cortex may play an important role in pain and episodic memory retrieval.

A close association with the limbic system means the collective workings of the cingulate gyrus are believed to be influential in linking behavioural outcomes to motivation (i.e. action + positive emotional response = learning). This part of the brain is therefore also believed to play an important role in disorders such as depression.

The Lateral Postcentral Gyrus

The lateral postcentral gyrus is another important and prominent structure reflexologists should become familiar with. It is situated in the parietal lobe of the brain, and the location of the primary somatosensory cortex; the main sensory receptive area for the sense of touch.

The Primary Somatosensory Cortex

The primary somatosensory cortex acts to ensure tactile representation in the brain is arranged in an orderly fashion, starting from the toe (at the top of the cerebral hemisphere) and working down to the mouth (located at the bottom). The map of this brain space is called the somatosensory **homunculus**.

The expanse of cortex within the homunculus allocated to represent each body part is not necessarily proportional to the size of the organ or part, but more seems to be arranged to represent the *density* of tactile receptors associated with any particular part of the body. In addition researchers believe there may be some overlap in the homunculus representing areas.

Neurons from primary somatosensory cortex send axons to the secondary somatosensory cortex, cortical motor areas, brain stem and spinal cord.

"The brain areas responsible for the perception of touch on the hands in the somatosensory homunculus are mostly located in the front if those areas responsible for hand movements in the motor homunculus. (Gallace & Spence, 2014)

Finally, it is important to note each cerebral hemisphere of the primary somatosensory cortex demonstrates tactile representation for the opposite (contralateral) side of the body.

The Secondary Somatosensory Cortex

The secondary somatosensory cortex is located in the lower parietal lobe. This part of the brain receives connections bilaterally from both the primary somatosensory cortex and also the thalamus. Neurons from the secondary somatosensory cortex in turn send axons back to the primary somatosensory cortex and association cortex, motor cortex and insular cortex.

Somatosensory Association Areas

In essence the somatosensory association areas give meaning to sensations. Each primary sensory area projects to a different association area. The association areas are responsible for higher mental and emotional processes, including learning and memory.

These areas of the brain draw upon stored memories to give meaning to present sensations, such as recognising particular sounds, or the feeling of a certain item in your pocket. It is possible these areas may also be associated with the manner in which the individual *perceives* the person providing the touch.

Neurogenesis

Neurogenesis refers to the manner in which the growing brain is populated with neurons. Researchers previously believed most of this process happened before birth and was completed through early childhood. However, scientists now understand more about this process of modification in the brain and confirm it is an ongoing and fluid process. Neurogenesis and neuroplasticity allow the brain to adapt to varying demands placed on it throughout life.

Communications in the Brain

The brain contains a network of at least 90 billion neurons, with each neuron a complex information-processing device in its own right. Neurons receive messages to their body from other neurons through short extensions called dendrites, at sophisticated junctions called synapses. Messages are transmitted to other neurons via long slender fibres called axons. Each message, or impulse is measured at around 0.1volt - lasts one to two thousandth of a second - and travels at 480kph (300mph). Glial cells outnumber neurons in the brain by 50:1. As well as being responsible for maintaining chemical balance in the brain, glial cells help neurons to wire together, or fuse, in the developing brain. Additionally, they support the adult brain, insulate axons, dispose of dead cells, recycle neurotransmitters, and finally help to protect the brain from infection.

Neurotransmitters

Impulses within the brain trigger the release of signalling transmitters called neurotransmitters. Neurotransmitters are released when nerve impulses arrive at synapses, and are responsible for conveying signals between neurons - either briefly *exciting* or *inhibiting* any electrical activity.

- **Excitatory neurotransmitters**: These neurotransmitters increase the likelihood that the neuron will fire an action potential. Neurotransmitters in this category include **epinephrine** and **norepinephrine**. Norepinehrine is responsible for stimulatory processes in the body and plays a role is producing epinephrine. This neurotransmitter is known to increase anxiety and cause mood dampening effects at elevated levels, as well as being associated with low energy, decreased focusing ability, and sleep problems. Epinephrine is known to be associated with stress and insomnia, and additionally plays a role in heart rate and blood pressure.

- **Inhibitory neurotransmitters**: These neurotransmitters decrease the likelihood that the neuron will fire an action potential. Balanced **serotonin** levels are required to ensure mood stabilisation and to balance the effect of excessive excitatory (stimulating) neurotransmitters. Serotonin also helps to regulate processes such as pain control, sleep cycles and food cravings (carbohydrates). Finally, low serotonin levels have been linked to lower levels of immunity. Stimulant medication and caffeine can also cause depletion of serotonin. **GABA** is often referred to as nature's *valium-like* substance and is produced to balance the effects of excitatory neurotransmitters.

- **Dopamine:** Considered both excitatory and inhibitory. Dopamine is the main focusing neurotransmitter. When dopamine levels are low it is possible to have problems with concentration and memory. Certain stimulants, such as caffeine can stimulate dopamine into the synapses, so that focus becomes improved, however, used consistently, this can also cause a depletion of dopamine.

Neurotransmitters range in size and are stored in tiny spheres called synaptic vesicles. Neurotransmitters act by binding to receptor proteins, with each protein finely tuned to receive a particular type of neurotransmitter.

Nerve Receptors in the Body

Specialised sensory receptors may be modified neurons, e.g., **photoreceptors** (vision) and **olfactory** receptors (smell), or modified epithelial cells, e.g., **taste** receptors and the **auditory** (hearing) and **vestibular** hair cells.

Proprioceptors provide the central nervous system with information about the movement of body parts in relation to other parts.

Interocepters respond to sensory stimuli from inside the body (internal body sensation), i.e., stomach pain, pinched spinal nerves, deep inflammation.

Exteroceptors respond to stimuli from the external environment and are located closest to the body surface.

Complex Interacting Systems

"The modern consensus is that while many functions are indeed associated with particular brain areas, each function nonetheless depends on interactions in widely distributed networks involving many different areas." (Seth, 2014)

Researchers are now clear in stating that no one specific area of the brain is entirely responsible for any single given function. Rather neuroscientists inform us whilst there is undoubtedly functional specialisation existing within parts of the brain, any given action is only made possible because of complex networks and mechanisms within different brain regions working together to coordinate any response.

We can find a good example of this response complexity in an area of the brain called the *amygdala*. The amygdala is a bundle of neurons (nuclei) approximately the size of a walnut buried deep in the medial lobe of the cerebral cortex. The amygdala represents an important structure within the limbic system.

The Limbic System

The limbic system describes a group of functionally and anatomically interconnected nuclei and cortical structures located in a portion of the cerebral cortex, folded deep within the lateral sulcus (the fissure separating the temporal lobe from the parietal and frontal lobes). The nuclei associated with the limbic system help to regulate autonomic and endocrine function, particularly in response to emotional stimuli. Additionally the system is associated with arousal, motivation, the olfactory system, and some parts are believed crucial to memory function.

The limbic system comprises several brain structures:

Amygdala: located in the **medial temporal lobes.** A bundle of nuclei involved in emotional responses and hormonal secretion. The amygdala, along with the hippocampus, also plays an important role in memory. The amygdala is responsible for determining which memories should be stored, and where they should be stored in the brain. Researchers believe this determination may be based on the strength of the emotional impact linked to any given event.

Cingulate Gyrus: an arched convolution located next to the corpus **callosum,** separated from it by the **sulcus of the corpus callosum.** The cingulate gurus is heavily involved with sensory input concerning emotion, pain, and the regulation of aggressive behaviour, as well as driving the conscious response to unpleasant experience. The area is linked to fear, and the prediction (and avoidance) of negative consequences, thus it works to encourage orientation of the individual away from negative stimuli. This form of learning is an important feature of memory.

Fornix: a fibrous band of nerve fibers connecting the hippocampus to the hypothalamus.

Hippocampus: located in the **medial temporal lobes**. The hippocampus is a bit like the brains memory indexer. The hippocampus sends memories to the appropriate part of the brain for long-term storage and retrieves memory when necessary. The hippocampus is also involved in spacial awareness.

Thalamus: part of the diencephalon located at the top of the **brain stem.** The thalamus are bundle of neurons (nuclei) heavily interconnected with specific areas of the **cerebral cortex** and are believed to act as sensory relay areas, connecting sensory receptors (apart from olfaction) with the cortex.

Hypothalamus: part of the diencephalon located at the top of the **brain stem**. The hypothalamus plays a major role in regulating hormones, the pituitary gland, body temperature, the adrenal glands, and finally it also represents an important emotional centre.

To demonstrate: - Scientists have discovered when the **amygdala** is damaged or removed from the brain individuals report a dampening of experienced emotion, and more specifically a loss of *fear*. Attempting to assess the loss caused by damage to the individuals responsive experience might only be appreciated through first comprehending the collective structures in the brain involved in translating the amygdala's function to a visceral and emotional reality.

Think for a moment what it would mean to lose your sense of fear?

- Fear may be commonly defined as an emotion, but does that definition isolate fear within a cognitive thinking category only? What about the accompanying physiological responses to fear? Think of the autonomic responses and the impact of the fight or flight response?

- Now think about decision making with no active sense of fear? In good measure fear helps to keep us safe? What happens when that safely gate is gone?

- How might fear and anticipation be related?

As we begin to appreciate more fully the complexities involved in this example it becomes increasingly transparent the *network* connected to the amygdala, and not the structure itself, is responsible for our ability to really *feel* and *experience* fear, viscerally and emotionally. Understanding more about the damaged brain permits us to appreciate the overall complex collective work of the brain's many nuclei and structures in manifesting any particular sensory experience.

On reflection it would appear quite impossible to isolate one single area of the brain as entirely responsible for any specific response. Rather, it is the co-ordinated action of many parts that defines the whole response. Apparently, evolution decided it would be best if our brain listened to, and communicated with, our minds and our bodies simultaneously.

Now, with this concept in mind, try to consider the wider impact of a reflexology intervention. As you interact with your clients feet, so too you are interacting with their brain. That unique brain exists within a conscious human being and their perception of you is heavily influencing the manner in which they, and their bodies, are responding to your touch.

Here Come the Hormones!

The brain is the main control deck upon which decisions are made in the body. The manner in which the brain carries out many of its co-ordinated responses is intimately associated with the functions of the **endocrine system**.

The Hypothalamus

The hypothalamus transmits sensory messages from the body to the brain - and from the brain to the body; effectively utilising the pituitary gland as the connection between the nervous system and the endocrine system. The hypothalamus is connected to the pituitary gland by a band of nervous tissue called the infundibulum.

The Pituitary Gland

The pituitary gland (or hypophysis) is located in the centre of the skull, inferior to the hypothalamus and posterior to the bridge of the nose. The pituitary gland links the **nervous** and **endocrine** systems of the body, and is responsible for secreting several hormones affecting growth, sexual development, metabolism, and human reproduction.

The pituitary gland sits well protected within a small cavity located in the sphenoid bone of the skull known as the hypophyseal fossa.

The Fight or Flight Response

The fight or flight response is an innate acute stress response controlled by the hypothalamus. Some communications in the brain lead to conscious thought and action, whilst others produce autonomic responses such as fight or flight. The aim of the response is to keep us safe, and it is therefore a vital part of our most basic human survival mechanisms. The mind and feelings or fear and anxiety trigger the fight or flight response in reaction to that experienced as *real* or *perceived* danger. When danger is perceived the hypothalamus activates two systems - the sympathetic nervous system and the adrenal-cortical system. The sympathetic nervous system uses the nerve pathways to initiate reactions in the body, and the adrenal-cortical system uses the bloodstream. It is the combined effects of these two systems that produce the fight or flight response.

The involvement of the sympathetic nervous system ensures the body speeds up ready to take action. Heart rate and blood pressure rise accordingly, whilst signals are sent to muscles warning them to be alert. The stress hormones adrenaline and nonadrenaline are released into the bloodstream by the adrenal gland. The hypothalamus releases corticotropin-releasing factor (CRF) to the pituitary gland, thus activating the adrenal-cortical system. In turn the pituitary gland secretes ACTH (adrenocorticotropic hormone) which then moves through the bloodstream, arriving at the adrenal cortex where it activates the release of other hormones designed to help the body prepare to deal with the threat.

High levels of cortisol, the body's primary stress hormone, increase, for example, levels of glucose in the bloodstream and enhance the brain's use of glucose. In addition, cortisol in the bloodstream increases availability of anti-inflammatory substances responsible for tissue repair. Finally, cortisol acts to curb any function deemed as nonessential in the fight or flight situation. Cortisol is also therefore involved in altering immune system response, and suppressing the function of digestive system, the reproductive system, and the growth processes.

"Stress can lead to changes in the serum level of many hormones including glucocorticoids, catecholamines, growth hormone and prolactin. Some of these changes are necessary for the fight or flight response to protect oneself. Some of these stressful responses can lead to endocrine disorders like Graves' disease, gonadal dysfunction, psychosexual dwarfism and obesity. Stress can also alter the clinical status of many preexisting endocrine disorders such as precipitation of adrenal crisis and thyroid storm." (Ranabir & Reetu, 2011)

Mind Influencing Body

"Emotion involves the entire neuraxis of brain stem, limbic areas, and superior cortex, as well as visceral and motor processes of the body. It encompasses psychosomatic networks of molecular communication along the nervous system, immune system, and endocrine system. On an emotional level, emotion involves attention and evaluation or appraisal, as well as affective feeling."(Thompson, 2007)

One important experiment helping to clarify emotional reactions to stress factors (Schacher & Singer, 1962) involved injecting volunteers with adrenaline, while an actor close by behaved either angrily or euphorically. One group of participants were informed prior to the event of the possible arousing effects of adrenaline. The other group were not informed.

The participants belonging to the informed group did *not* experience any associated emotional response, whilst the participants belonging to the *uninformed* group reported experiencing similar feelings of anger and euphoria.

This particular experiment allowed researchers to suggest a *'felt'* or experienced emotion depends entirely on the manner in which the brain *interprets* the changes occurring in the body.

"It is now widely accepted that emotions are deeply dependant on how the brain and body react to each other." (Seth, 2014)

Interventions such as tactile affection can also impact physiological variables such as blood pressure and heart rate. This concept was investigated by Grewen et al., (2003). In this study participants were allocated to one of two groups. The contact group underwent a 10-minute handholding session while watching a romantic video, followed by a 20-second hug. The no contact group rested for 10-minutes, and 20-seconds. Following this both sets of participants were asked to perform a stressful public speaking event. The results revealed those individuals receiving pre-stressor tactile contact demonstrated significantly lower systolic and diastolic blood pressure and heart rate increases than the no contact group.

Note: It is important to remember in a study such as this it would be impossible to separate any reaction related to tactile intervention from the larger global context in which the touch is experienced. This means it is vitally important to consider other influencing factors. In this study specifically, factors worth consideration would include the touch being provided by a close trusted partner in full visual sight, and the impact of the video tape, etc.

Epigenetics

"While genes certainly affect brain function, the fact they can be influenced by their environment frees our behaviour from a rigid genetic determinism as the brain's genetic machinery responds adaptively to changing circumstances." (Seth, 2014)

Epigenetic literally means 'above genetics'. Epigenetic control is related to how environmental signals control the activity of genes. It relates to the phenomena whereby genetically identical cells can express their genes differently; a phenomenon that changes the final outcome of a cell without changing the underlying DNA sequence. Put simply, a bladder cell is always destined to be a bladder cell, but under certain environmental circumstances it may emerge as an *inflammatory* bladder cell.

The field of Epigenetics is responsible for scientifically establishing that DNA blueprints handed down at birth are not absolute or set in stone. Rather, the study of epigenetic's has helped to highlight that environmental influences, including nutrition, stress and emotional states can modify genes *without* changing their blueprint, and that those modifications can then be passed on to offspring and future generations.

Epigenetic Change

"Genes are simply molecular blueprints used in the construction of cells, tissues, and organs. The environment acts as a "contractor" who reads and engages those genetic blueprints and is ultimately responsible for the characteristics of a cell's life." (Lipton, 2008)

When a neural circuit detects a consistent potential threatening sensory stimulus, strengthened circuit connections become necessary to help sustain and enhance states of vigilance. To achieve this stance signals are dispatched from synapses to their central nuclei, where the DNA contained within activates appropriate threat response genes. In turn, newly made synapse-reinforcing proteins (now ready to receive their associated neurotransmitters) are bonded to the synapses that ordered the response initially.

In depressive disorders for instance researchers believe:

"chronic stress as an epigenetic factor changes the gene regulation pattern by interrupting the Dopamine signalling mechanism. (Mariam & Sobhsni, 2013)

A review (Stankiewicz et al., 2013) examining how epigenetic influences might be associated with stress adaptations in the brain, concluded;

"that specific epigenetic mechanisms in the CNS are involved in the stress response."

The study also identified that the characteristics of epigenetic stress responses depends on multitude of factors. Other epigenetic studies have looked at how environmental influences can impact health more specifically. One study (Wilson, 2008) investigated epigenetic regulation of gene expression in the human inflammatory response, and its relevance to common diseases. The study concluded:

"The importance of the epigenome in the pathogenesis of common human diseases is likely to be as significant as that of traditional genetic mutations.

A study linked to asthma (Ji & Khurana Hershey, 2012) looked at genetic and epigenetics influences in response to environmental particulate matter. Finding demonstrated:

"Epidemiologic evidence supports that environmental exposures in childhood affect susceptibility to disease later in life, supporting the belief that epigenetic changes can affect ongoing development and promote disease long after the environmental exposure has ceased.

A review (Biola et al., 2011) considering how environmental triggers and epigenetic deregulation might be linked to autoimmune disorders stated:

"The breakdown of epigenetic regulation is now known to play a key role in the development of diseases."

Several studies have looked at the impact of epigenetic factors regarding sub-fertility (see also sub-fertility chapter).

"Increasing evidence suggests that genetic and environmental factors can have negative effects on epigenetic processes controlling implantation, placentation and fetal growth." (Dada, et al., 2012)

Note: The beneficial impact of reflexology in inflammatory, autoimmune, and sub-fertility conditions to name but a few, is certainly well evidenced antidotally. In the future, as we come to learn more about the wider impact of sustained stress and anxiety on the human body, we may also find the requirement for therapeutic interventions such a reflexology becomes more pronounced.

The Default Mode Network

"Activity within the default mode network is reduced during focus upon an externally directed task, and more defined during states of wakeful rest, mind wandering, introspection, or inwardly directed attention. This network includes medial parts pre-frontal and temporal lobes and the posterior cingulate cortex. (Seth, 2014)

Stress responses in the body are designed to stand down once the threat has passed. The opposing default state occurs when the body is no longer in perceived danger, and the functioning of the autonomic nervous system has returned to normal. The body thus moving from a state of physiological arousal, to a state of default where the blood pressure, heart rate, digestive functioning and hormonal levels all stabilise. Without any specific task to perform (resting brain state) researchers have discovered the brain is actually almost as active as when occupied. However, during such resting times a different set of default brain regions displays activity, rather than those areas associated more specifically with task-related activity. The default mode network is defined by co-ordinated activity over a wide range of cortical areas located primarily along the 'cortical midline', where the two hemispheres of the brain meet.

"This network was originally identified as a set of brain regions consistently deactivated during tasks that require externally oriented attention. Later imaging studies showed that this network is active during internally focused cognitive processes such as moral decision making and planning of future behaviour and also that it can reliably be identified during resting conditions." (Van Dijk & Drzezga, 2014)

Note: Arousal refers to an internal state of vigilance, alertness, or cognitive information processing.

Scientists believe the default state to be heavily associated with day-dreaming and spontaneous thinking, and that increased activity in this part of the brain can lead to higher levels of personal insight and states of creativity. Researchers have gathered some limited evidence regarding the default state in the infant brain, and a larger body of evidence in the 9-12 year old age group. Scientists also believe the default network may undergo changes as we grow older.

"Brain functional network organisations are dynamically optimised for a higher level of information integration in the fully conscious awake state, and that the default-mode network plays a pivotal role in information integration for maintaining conscious awareness." (Uehara et al., 2014)

In terms of trying to understand how this mind-wandering state might be beneficial to emotional health more specifically, let us momentarily turn our attention to the field of non-directive play therapy. Children who have been severely traumatised often lack an inner world of imagination and a natural ability to play. Researchers believe this may be due to disruptions in the *cingulate gyrus*. As a trainee counsellor I was fortunate to complete part of the clinical component of my degree working with emotionally vulnerable infant school children. Non-directive play therapy is perhaps unlike any other form of counselling. The intervention is entirely person-centred, meaning the children set the tone of the sessions and hold autonomy over how they utilise the play therapy room. In essence, the therapist, within the confines of the therapeutic relationship, is accompanying the child on their play journey - however that may manifest.

The value for children in imaginative, creative play is astonishingly powerful, and quite a phenomenon to witness personally. Children generally seem more at ease with stepping into this relaxed, intuitive part of their being and through accessing this more creative, imaginative state are somehow able to *integrate* their existing emotional content. It is entirely possible to work with a child over many months using play therapy without the issue involving the child being verbalised within the sessions, however, the therapeutic process seems to allow the children to manage and sort through their feelings and emotions.

For instance, sandbox work is perhaps one of the most powerful interventions in non-directive play therapy. Often this form of play does not centre around a 'story', as such, in the manner it might when the play involves the doll's house or the car mat, but instead, during sand play the child might appear to focus on the *feel* of sand running through their fingers, or sometimes the child might silently bury a toy deep in the sand, over and over again. During this type of play the child is processing emotionally on a deep level, and so perhaps this deeper introspective state might be most likened to the adult default mind-wandering state.

"The assumption is that given the opportunity to express themselves freely, children will reach solutions and resolve their own emotional difficulties themselves, using play experiences and their therapists to do so." (Wilson & Ryan, 2005)

Because adults have the tendency to be cognitively busy and ever occupied it is possible they are visiting the default mind wandering state much less frequently than perhaps they should. In any conscious situation the brain is required to access the memory to utilise already stored information, in order to make more informed decisions. Forward projecting, planning, strategising, organising and worrying all require the involvement of the more cognitive parts of the human brain. The default state however, seems to be a place where the mind is disconnected from specific tasking, and instead turns to filing and organising our emotional content and memories. From this place of unfocused introspection the brain can also signal for stabilisation of the nervous and endocrine system, thus encouraging the manifestation of a wider state of homeostasis.

Touch in Counselling and Psychotherapy

Despite some of the clear psychological and physiological well-being benefits associated with interpersonal touch the concept remains a rather thorny issue in the counseling and psychotherapy world; with most instances of touch generally discouraged. In fact, studies within the talking therapy field demonstrate a concern among talking therapists that instances of interpersonal touch might be perceived as *"inappropriate"* (Rutter, 1989); (Stenzel & Rupert, 2004); (Galton, 2006). A recent detailed analysis of touch in the field states the most common forms of touch remain as *"handshakes and hugs."* (Williams et al., 2011).

The Meditative Brain State

The practice of meditation is increasingly demonstrating profoundly positive effects on the human brain. Scientists have been able to confirm for example, those individuals involved in long term meditation tend to display shrunken amygdala's, (*linked to states of anxiety and fear*), as well as an enlarged prefrontal cortex (*linked to cognitive processing and intelligence*). Meditation is also believed to improve a wide range of tasks, including attention, working memory, spacial processing tasks, visual and tactile perception, and is even believed to reduce the requirement for sleep.

The Feet

The feet are among the most nerve-rich parts of the body. When standing and walking the soles of feet are the body parts in direct touch with the environment. Sensory information is used to protect the feet from injury, to make adjustments in the gait in order to protect the joints of the body, and to maximise efficiency in movements.

"The tactile receptors on the soles of our feet provide us (or rather our brains) with a constant source of information about the characteristics of the surface we happen to be walking on; that is, whether it remains constant, such as when we stand waiting at the bus-stop, or whether it changes continuously, such as on the deck of a boat out sailing on

a choppy sea. This information is constantly integrated with vestibular cues regarding the position of our body in three dimensional (3D) space." (Gallace & Spence, 2014)

It takes only milliseconds for sensory information from the feet to reach the brain, and in turn for the brain to respond by making adjustments to muscles in the legs, back and arms.

Deposits in Reflex Areas

Dr Jesus Manzanares, a Spanish based reflexology researcher, engaged in a study involving taking biopsies from the feet of three adult volunteers to determine anatomical characteristics and tissue composition. Biopsies were taken from both non-deposit tissue and from reflex areas containing deposits associated with the stomach, lumbar and thymus reflex areas. The study concluded:

"Deposits are a mixture of organic composition as opposed to previous theory of inorganic matter calcification, crystals or toxins."

Biopsy Results:

Non-Deposit Tissue	Deposit Tissue
8% nervous fibers	42% nervous tissue
27% vascular elements	28% vascular elements
65% connective tissue	30% connective tissue

Dr Manzanares believes the results of his investigations support the concept of a relationship between reflexology and neurological system.

Note: This is an unpublished study. For more detailed information please visit Dr Manzanares webpage directly.

The Reflexology Space

"Therapists using touch in the form of reflexology may not consciously be within a psychodynamic contract, but the effect on self-image is likely to have some potency and subsequent health benefits." (Mackereth, 2011).

A study carried out by Christie's NHS Foundation, Manchester, (Mackereth et al., 2009) analysed taped transcripts of the verbal interactions occurring during reflexology sessions.

The research highlighted numerous examples of client originated enquiries occurring during the sessions. The study suggests clients seem to be gaining some form of therapeutic benefit from the wider reflexology environment, and feel able to talk openly with their therapist. The study demonstrated:

"Reflexology provided opportunities for 48 out of the 50 participants to share worries and concerns".

Similarly, (Gambles, Crooke, & Wilkinson, 2002) utilised semi-structured questionnaires to attempt to highlight some of the wider subjective existential benefits of receiving reflexology. Some of the statements provided in the study appear to confirm to the suggestion that reflexology, far from being identified as physical pressure therapy alone, seems also to contain an element identified as *relational* in essence:

"Being able to discuss my illness with caring and friendly staff"

"I just talked which was also very helpful"

"I had so much on my mind"

"The (therapist) was so helpful and caring"

"She helped me with advice"

Peter Mackereth (2011) believes *physiological* changes can occur as a consequence of *psychological* processes in reflexology, and given the complexity of the package these are likely to be working in '*synergy*'. Mackereth goes on to state reflexology provides space for:

"Psychological support and nurturing of the body."

A recent systematic literature review (McCullough et al., 2014) analysed existing data available from RCTs (randomised controlled trails) where investigation focused upon the physiological and biochemical changes associated with reflexology, and stated:

"a range of positive effects can be attributed to the treatment, specifically a reduction in stress parameters." and that; *"reflexology should be promoted for any medical condition where stress is contraindicated."*

In a randomised controlled trial (Bagheri-Nesami et al., 2014) 80 patients received foot reflexology on their left foot 20 min a day for 4 days, while the control group was given a gentle foot rub with oil for one minute. Anxiety was measured using the short-form of the Spielberger State-Trait Anxiety Inventory and the Visual Analogue Scale-Anxiety. The study demonstrated:

"Both measurement instruments confirmed a significant decrease in anxiety following the foot reflexology massage."

and,

"The significant decrease in anxiety in the experimental group following the foot reflexology massage supports the use of this complementary therapy technique for the relief of anxiety.

In a Korean study (Jang & Kim, 2009) researchers studied the effects of self administered reflexology in middle-aged menopausal women. The study concluded:

"Reflexology may be an effective nursing intervention in reducing perceived stress, fatigue and blood circulation".

Another study (Quattrin, et al., 2006) examined the effectiveness of reflexology in reducing anxiety among hospitalised cancer patients, concluding reflexology, in combination with other treatments:

"Can help (patients) feel better and also cope with their disease".

Interestingly, a small quantitative research project (Trousdell & Uphoff-Chmielnic, 1997) looked at the efficiency of delivering reflexology and person-centred counselling *'concomitantly'* over the same time period indicated:

"Client's receiving both therapies moved to significantly more positive psychological posture and physical well-being within a shorter time than expected."

A study (McVicar et al., 2007) examining the effect of reflexology on anxiety, salivary cortisol and melatonin secretion concluded:

"Considering the connection between stress/anxiety and well being, the effects of reflexology may have beneficial outcomes for patients."

Other Reflexology Research

There are now over 150 published reflexology studies, the greater majority of which originating from within the clinical sector. Just one recent example is Dalal et al., (2014) who looked at the of efficacy of reflexology in managing patients with diabetic neuropathy using outcome measures related to pain reduction, glycemic control, nerve conductivity, and thermal and vibration sensitivities. The study concluded:

"Reflexology group showed more improvements in all outcome measures than those of control subjects with statistical significance. Conclusion. This study exhibited the

efficient utility of reflexology therapy integrated with conventional medicines in managing diabetic neuropathy."

Reflexology and the Brain

A Japanese study (Naoki et al, 2013) utilised fMRI to examine related brain activity in recipients receiving specific reflexology stimulation to the eye reflex point/area when compared to a sham point (shoulder). Findings demonstrated:

"a robust relationship exists between neural processing of somatosensory percepts for reflexological stimulation and the tactile sensation of a specific reflex area in the left middle postcentral gyrus, the area to which tactile sensation to the face projects, as well as in the postcentral gyrus contralateral foot representation area."

Another study (Sliz et al., 2012) used fMRI to investigate the neurophysiological effects of different types of massage in healthy adults. Participants were assigned to one of four groups; Swedish massage, reflexology, massage with an object, or the resting control group. In this study the right foot was massaged, and then massaged while participants completed a cognitive task:

"Interestingly, the reflexology massage condition selectively affected the retrosplenial/posterior cingulate in the resting state, whereas massage with the object augmented the BOLD response in this region during the cognitive task performance.

*Note: Evidence suggests the **retrosplenial cortex** might play a role in the interaction between emotion and episodic memory. (Maddock, 1999)*

In another study (Nakamaru et al., 2008), individuals were subjected to functional magnetic resonance imaging fMRI of the brain. Three reflexology points were stimulated: the eye, the shoulder and the small intestine. reflexology points were chosen because of the distance between each other and therefore their distinction on the projection area of the somatosensory homunculus. Stimulation was applied using a wooden stick, via auditory instruction (using headphones) from the imaging technician. The experimenter held of the instep of the left foot while applying stimulation.

The study demonstrated the eye specific point displayed most activity in the middle part of the left post central gyrus. The small intestine showed most activity in the superior part of the left post central gyrus shoulder stimulation did not appear to be significant, but showed tendency for increased local activity in the superior part of the right post central gyrus (*this might be explained because of a reduction in the saturation of sensory nerves associated with the shoulder in general*).

Normally when the left side of the body is stimulated in MRI studies then the right side of the brain is activated, but in this study the left side stimulation results in left brain activation, based on the results obtained from the eye and small intestine. This finding seems to support the reflexology tenet that left side stimulation results in left side activation.

In an earlier study (Tang et al., 2006) researchers used fMRI to compare brain activity using reflexology and electro-stimulation when stimulation was given to the reflex area identified as the adrenal gland point, and the acupuncture point identified at K1 (both located in the same area). Researchers found brain activity in both instances was:

"*mostly localised at insula region.*"

Note: In fMRI studies such as these it is important to remain mindful of the very artificial environment in which the experiments are taking place. Clearly, these results offer only a small glimpse into the possible brain activity that might be associated with more normal forms of reflexology practice.

Summary

"Anybody who has been seriously engaged in scientific work of any kind realises that over the entrance to the gates of the temple of science are written the words: Ye must have faith." - Max Planck

Tactile receptors and nerve fibers were first identified in human beings around twenty years ago, and it has only been in the last five years their role in a number of human behaviours has started to be investigated. Modern neuroscience equipment is rapidly offering scientists entry to an exciting world of possibility and discovery. The neurological structures highlighted within this article represent, *for the moment*, the areas of the brain most likely to be involved in the overall reflexology experience. These are the areas of the brain representing the complex systems related to both the manner in which our brains interpret and react to instances of interpersonal touch, and also the areas of the brain associated with filing and sorting emotional content, and memory.

Whilst scientists are only at the beginning of their journey in studying the most complex entity on the planet - the human brain, they do seem fairly sure regarding one thing involving interpersonal touch:

"It is not really important what a person is actually feeling, but what a person believes they are feeling." (Gallace & Spence, 2014)

Scientists tell us tactile experience is entirely influenced by the individual's social perception of the person providing the touch, and refer to this phenomenon as the '*Midas Touch.*' Indeed, touch researchers openly acknowledge the *Midas touch* is extremely difficult to reproduce in mediated test environments (Gallace & Spence, 2014). After all, compare the average touch experiment with the real experience and length of a full reflexology session. Consider the inviting therapy room, the client wrapped safely in warm blanket and the presence of a friendly, caring face? In terms of reflexology the *Midas touch* may well emerge as simply humanity in a therapy room.

"I wouldn't be surprised to observe that reflexology works well if delivered by a human being but not at all if the same pattern of stimulation is provided by a mechanical stimulator." (Alberto Gallace, via email communication)

So what does this mean for the art of reflexology? Firstly, I believe it means we need to be patient and give science time to do what science does best - and that is to explore. Considering how much has been discovered about the brain, interpersonal touch, and emotion in just five years, I very much doubt we will have too much longer before we can really start to make sense of what might be occurring in reflexology. I hope in the meantime this chapter provides some informed clues as to how our wider interventions might be impacting clients, as well as hinting towards the some of the directions reflexology research may take in the future. I also believe the time has come to highlight more clearly the difference between *justifying* the modality, and attempting to justify our more rounded therapeutic work. Some of the information presented here clearly demonstrates the brains default state is closely associated with homeostasis of the mind and body. In this respect the underlying principles of reflexology seem utterly sound - *relaxation is profoundly good for the mind and body.*

As we start to contextualise reflexology in the manner it is more often practiced; with vulnerable client groups, often craving emotional support and advice, it also becomes clear there are *other* aspects relating to our practice that might require our professional attention. Professional practitioners should always be driven by an ethical principle centred upon providing each individual client with high levels of care and appropriate information. Practitioners should be ready to empathically acknowledge a clients tears and frustrations, and poised to keep safe their emotionally vulnerable clients, in addition to providing appropriate information where necessary. In private practice, where money is exchanging hands, this stance is particularly important. Part of my role as a therapist is to support my client in their quest to feel better, in as efficient a manner as possible.

Later in the book some of the case study examples will highlight this important concept. Much of my work is soundly underpinned by the information I provide to clients. Marc's example (interstitial cystitis case study) demonstrates the information I was able to offer presented a new context in which my client was able to consider his internal reactions to his experience, and wider environment - *outside* of the confines of our weekly reflexology sessions. This stance certainly does not lessen the impact of reflexology, nor does it detract from its positive therapeutic impact, rather it perhaps more clearly demonstrates the difference between the modality - and the reality of the type of therapeutic work undertaken more generally. Many reflexology clients are increasingly required to deal with mounting levels of continuous stress and pressure, certainly an unfortunate side effect of our hurried, competitive, driven society. It certainly would seem unwise these days to display as weak, fearful, or indecisive. Instead, many clients are quietly encouraged to dismiss their internal emotional states, and levels of personal exhaustion, and simply plough on. Cognitively smart and high functioning human beings may be, but that certainly does not mean our emotional states are unimportant, particularly when considering the subject of human health and well-being. On the contrary, as scientific evidence clearly demonstrates, human emotional states are intrinsically connected to our states of physical health, and indeed in turn, to our internal perception of health.

"Repression – disassociating emotions from awareness and relegating them to the unconscious realm – disorganises and confuses our physiological defences." (Mate, 2003)

The human body and brain are deeply complex and highly detailed. The multi-dimensional impact of the supportive reflexology package is also complex and detailed. I believe reflexology may stand proud as one of the few complementary therapies capable of impacting human beings across several interrelated dimensions of real and phenomenological experience. Who knows? In the future reflexology may well come to define the very essence of the holistic phrase - *mind, body, soul*. In my mind it already does.

Relational Reflexology

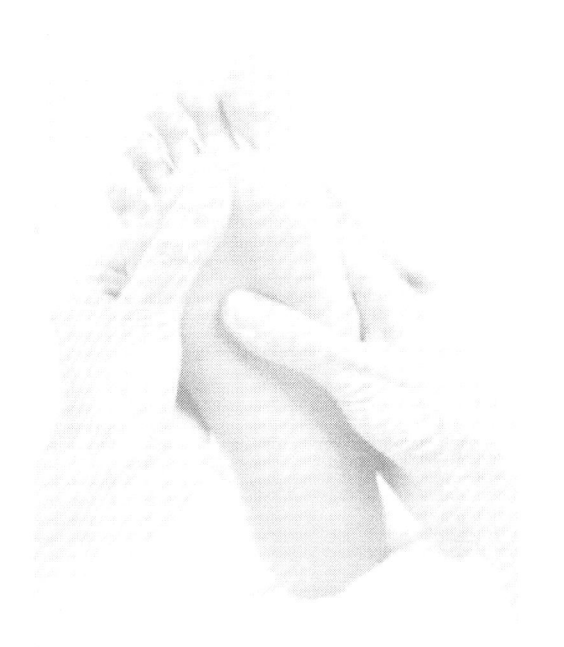

To Treat or Not to Treat, That is the Question
Fear and Contraindication in Reflexology

"I have been and still am a seeker, but I have ceased to question stars and books; I have begun to listen to the teaching my blood whispers to me."

- Hermann Hesse

I initially qualified in reflexology via one of the more overly cautious training bodies here in the U.K. Realistically, if I had continued to adhere to the 'rules' I was initially asked to follow, I probably would not still be in practice today. The list of contraindications promoted by the training provider doubled in size during my training, leaving frankly only the perfectly healthy individual open to freely access treatment.

A real deep fear of causing harm seems to exist in many of today's reflexology practitioners. In some cases this is initiated by the primary training body, and in other cases it can be attributed to a lack of practitioner experience, or self development. Some training bodies unfortunately seem to spend a great deal of time concentrating on application and technique alone, and not nearly enough time (if any) promoting the concept of holistic back engineering, or indeed exploring why reflexology might be impacting clients so positively(collectively this encourages the concept of working with the whole person). Nor do many training bodies promote an appropriate form of practitioner self development; one ultimately capable of instilling a heightened sense of practitioner self awareness, encouraging development of the internal supervisor. Unfortunately without the promotion of such concepts, as our awareness develops regarding the power of reflexology to promote more balanced health and wellbeing (often without really understanding why that might be), practitioners can also find they remain fearful that same power may be capable of causing harm to clients.

Ethical Decision Making

Remaining mindful of the limitations existing within the reflexology package, and indeed in our own professional competencies, is of course entirely ethical, but how might practitioners best define exactly where those ethical boundaries lie? The challenge for practitioners in ethical decision making is to balance our real and perceived fears and concerns against our knowledge and experience, ideally then arriving at a decision – *or a state of being* – where we feel comfortable in our ability to confidently meet the needs of our client. A good rule when making an ethical decision is where no clear path is illuminated, one should take the path that causes least harm. Put simply, if you are unsure, do not proceed.

Beneficence is an ethical principle most connected with applying therapeutic skills to help people. It relates to and might be defined as actions which are taken to benefit another.

In reflexology the duty of beneficence must be considered together with its converse duty, that of **non-maleficence**, which is the concept of ensuring no one is hurt. This principle should ensure that any risks involved are proportionate to the benefits.

Back Engineering Holistically – When Common Sense and Knowledge Say Yes!

I was contacted by Sue, 31 weeks pregnant, diagnosed with Obstetric cholestasis (OC). Obstetric cholestasis is a condition of the liver, specifically a reduced flow of bile from the bile ducts in the liver. Liver enzymes, and in particular bile salts, leak into the bloodstream causing symptoms (severe itching across the body, but often most pronounced in the hands and feet, tiredness, and understandable emotional distress). Fairly commonly, women with OC are induced at 37 weeks gestation - due to a slight increased risk of stillbirth. Sue was determined to avoid induction. Sue was under the care of a consultant obstetrician and her bloods were being checked weekly. I was certainly initially cautious about engaging, but after researching the condition I agreed to the work. I know from experience reflexology can certainly promote better circulation, which in turn can support liver function, and I was also confident reflexology support might help with my clients feeling of frustration and obvious distress. I did however make it clear to Sue, if her bloods test results remained outside normal range at 36 weeks, she *must* follow her consultants advice regarding induction.

I did not ask for written or verbal permission from the consultant, or the GP. In fact, I am often a little perplexed by the concept a medical doctor might be expected to know more about the impact of reflexology than me – the professional practitioner, or indeed that they might welcome endless enquires from unsure, insecure complementary therapists. Undoubtedly there are situations where it is in the client's best interests to inform the GP or consultant about the inclusion of reflexology, but that is not the same as asking for permission to proceed.

Sue and I agreed on a plan of action together.

- I would administer reflexology twice weekly

- Sue agreed to steep her feet in hot water, and to body brush daily to further improve circulation.

- Sue also agreed to start consuming an additive and preservative free diet, and to avoid tap water.

- We discussed Sue's feelings of frustration regarding the potential induction – an important element to cover because of the TCM link between liver energy and the emotions of anger and agitation.

- Sue agreed to engage in more instances of self care – including regular guided meditations, additional periods of rest, and trying to remain mindful of her emotional state.

Sue's itching subsided within a week, and by 36 weeks gestation all blood test results displayed within normal range. Sue was able to experience the home birth she so desired at 41.5 weeks, supported by her medical team.

My initial fears regarding engaging with this particular client were reduced principally because of my existing A&P knowledge, and because of my confidence and trust in my therapeutic modality. I researched the condition fully, applied that information to my A&P knowledge, and then to my knowledge of TCM, before arriving at a place where I felt confident to proceed. I explained my rationale for engaging in the work, and Sue and I worked together to invoke change.

When Fear Says No!

I received a telephone call from a gentleman in his early sixties, recently diagnosed with terminal lung cancer. During our telephone conversation this potential client disclosed his decision to refuse all offered medical treatment, believing instead complementary medicine held the potential to cure him entirely of the disease. As our conversation progressed I became aware of a huge weight of responsibility potentially being placed on my shoulders. His expectation regarding desired outcome felt heavy to me, and I can clearly recall feeling very uncomfortable and unsure. We talked for while and I tried hard to better manage his expectations regarding reflexology, whilst also encouraging him to consider re-engaging with his medical team. He was understandably angry and distressed regarding his diagnosis and completely adamant medical type cancer treatment was just not for him. In the end, and because of his emotional state, I respectfully declined to administer reflexology, explaining the potential weight of responsibility he was asking me to carry alone was just too much.

The decision I made in this case was based on my own feelings; an awareness that my own inner supervisor was not feeling at all confident. I was able to acknowledge my feelings and gut instinct, and from that place made my decision. This is the only client I have ever declined to work with.

Where Do The Boundaries Lie?

Of course there are times when practitioners need to be mindful regarding administering reflexology, for example, localised injury or infection, undiagnosed pain etc. Certainly also the presence of certain medication requires some additional consideration:

- **Blood thinners** (anticoagulants) such a Warfarin and Heparin. Probably the most important group of medication to be aware of. Only once INR (International Normalised Ratio) testing has confirmed the blood is clotting correctly should reflexology be administered. Until such a time reflexology is strictly contraindicated. A past history of clotting does not however contraindicate treatment.

- **Titrated medication** such as Thyroxine. Titration helps the body adapt slowly to certain medications, often reducing common side effects occurring when the individual first begins treatment. Titration additionally allows the physician to find an optimal dose for the individual. Whilst reflexology is not exclusively contraindicated in the presence of titrated medication, the practitioner should make the client aware of the potential impact of reflexology on the circulation, as this can sometimes mean bloods may require monitoring more regularly by the GP.

There are also certain client groups requiring additional consideration, again however, they are not entirely contraindicated:

- Pregnancy Group
- Sub-Fertility Group
- Cancer Care Group
- Palliative Care Group

Reflexology works subtly, on multi-dimensional levels, and always in line with the principles of homeostasis; helping to return the body to a place of calm, balance and equilibrium.

Homeostasis: Noun

1. *The tendency of a system especially the physiological system of higher animals, to maintain internal stability owing to the co-ordinated responses of its parts to any situation or stimulus that would tend to disturb its normal condition or function.*

2. *Psychology. A state of psychological equilibrium obtained when tension or a drive has been reduced or eliminated.*

Building Confidence in Practice

The key elements required to build practitioner confidence are:

- Practical Experience
- Good Levels of Appropriate Knowledge
- Reflective Practice
- Practitioner Self Awareness and the Development of the Inner Supervisor
- Peer Support and/or Professional Supervision
- Continuing Professional Development

'Physician, Heal Thyself'

So now let us perhaps imagine you have researched your client's condition fully and are content you understand the A&P involved. Perhaps you have asked for advice from a more experienced practitioner, or are fortunate enough to belong to a professional association where telephone advice is readily available, yet still find you feel unsure about proceeding? Why might this be?

Fear and anxiety can be strong emotions indeed. Sometimes we can be very aware of their presence, and at other times the feelings can be more sub-conscious in essence, and therefore more difficult to define. Practitioner self development can help to bring some of these sub-conscious emotions to a more transparent level. For many practitioners, engaging in reflective practice exercises and supervision, for example, can help with gaining more clarity regarding their fears. In other cases the practitioner may benefit from engaging directly with a supportive counsellor or psychotherapist.

The Wounded Healer

There is an interesting phenomenon occurs in professions where empathy is required and encouraged. Perhaps the best way to consider this phenomenon would be to enquire why you, the reader, trained as a reflexologist? The theme in essence relates to the concept of the *wounded healer*. Studies have demonstrated that in many cases individuals who have chosen to follow careers paths involving caring or helping as an element:

"often as children experienced loneliness, illness, bereavement or the need to look after others." (March-Smith, 2005)

Researchers have suggested that with these children the ability to empathise often develops to such an advanced degree in childhood, that as adults these individuals can then sometimes feel compelled to care for others and are therefore drawn towards more therapeutic professions.

"the presence of such a 'wound' in a healer gives them an excellent basis from which to understand and empathise with the wounds of clients." (McLoud, 1998)

Whilst certainly no assumption can be made that all complementary therapists possess such a inner wound, the concept does demonstrate the requirement for good levels of self awareness in all professional reflexology practitioners. Practitioners more aware of their inner motivations, thoughts and feelings are often:

- Better able to understand and regulate their emotional reactions.

- Better able to engage in appropriate levels of self care.

- Potentially in less danger of exhausting their own personal energy.

- Better able to maintain appropriate professional boundaries and to offer appropriate reflective responses.

- Better able to remain connected within the client's unique frame of reference.

Engaging with a supportive counsellor can feel like a wonderful journey of self exploration. There is absolutely no requirement to present for counselling with a particular problem or issue. The only requirement is a genuine desire to understand oneself more intimately, and with more clarity. Often increased levels of practitioner self-awareness can help to allay fears, helping us to grow in confidence and become more self directed and autonomous.

Summary

Every therapist is different. It is what makes human beings so wonderful – our uniqueness! There are some practitioners who will find their own rationale for practice and ethical decision making processes develop relatively easily, whilst for others the journey can seem bumpy and filled with caution and fear.

Our similarities as reflexologists lie in our desire to help others through the wonderfully therapeutic medium of reflexology. Our passion and desire to help others however, should always be accompanied by the ability to listen to our own internal drives and narrative.

Practitioner self development, ethical decision making and the concept of contraindication are inter-connected and related. Next time you feel fearful of causing harm, try to follow that fear to its source and examine more closely where it is coming from. Then take appropriate steps to balance your fear through education. All the very best therapists do.

Relational Reflexology

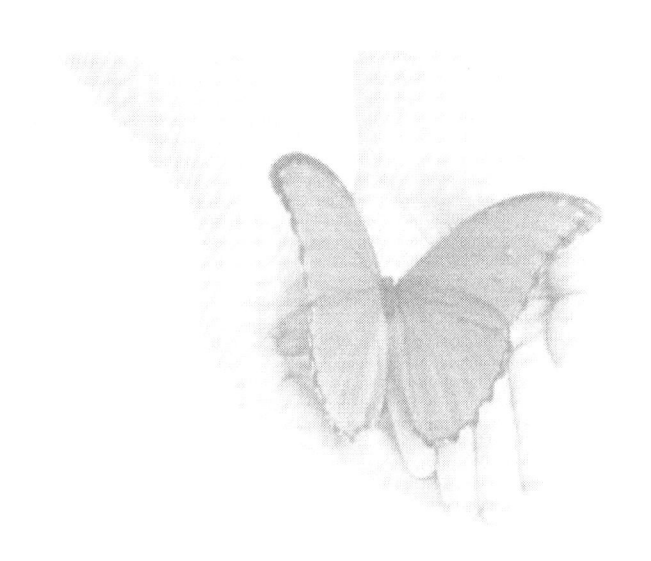

Philosophy and Well-Being in Reflexology

"Everything can be taken from a man or woman but one thing: the last of human freedoms to choose one's attitude in any given set of circumstances, to choose one's own way."

- Viktor Frankl

Mention the subject of philosophy to many people and it immediately conjures up images of serious men engaging in serious dialogue around very serious subjects. Whilst indeed philosophers across the ages have explored the "big" questions, such as the meaning of life, and the limitations of existential freedom, philosophical thinking can also be applied to the individual life, and so in many ways philosophy also underpins many forms of therapy.

The *Oxford Companion to Philosophy* defines philosophy as:

"Rationally critical thinking, of a more or less systematic kind about the general nature of the world (metaphysics or theory of existence), the justification of belief (epistemology or theory of knowledge) and the conduct of life (ethics or theory of value)" (Honderich, 1995)

The aim of any therapy is to help the client take control of aspects of their life. In reflexology more specifically we are focused upon helping the client to take control of their *'well-being'*. What defines well-being? Can well-being be contextualised as a universal truth, or might the concept be entirely unique to the individual? Is my definition of well-being likely to be similar to yours?

The Core Dimensions of Psychological Well-Being (PWB)

Ryff and Singers (2008) work, identifying the features of well-being was partially influenced by Carl Rogers (1951). Rogers previously discussed well-being in terms of the *"good life"* and the *"fully functioning person"*; an individual open to experience, trusting in his or her own organism, and leading a truly conscious life. There are five features of PWB:

- Self Acceptance
- Purpose in Life
- Environmental Mastery
- Positive Relationships
- Personal Growth and Autonomy

According to PWB health and well-being is best achieved when the individual is in possession of the appropriate psychological, social and/or physical resources required to meet any particular challenge. Should the individual be contending with more challenges than they have resources to deal with, then the metaphorical well-being seesaw can dip, rendering the individual feeling stressed, anxious or even depressed.

A strong sense of well-being is therefore best achieved through balancing a combination of physical, social, intellectual and emotional factors. This can be more clearly defined as a *holistic* definition of well-being.

Defining Individual Meaning

During the reflexology consultation period practitioners should ideally enquire of their client:

"What do you hope to gain from supportive reflexology?"

This is a crucially important question principally because it helps to clarify both the client's future expectation, and to give context to their present unique experience. Earlier in the book we briefly explored the concept of **phenomenology**. The goal of phenomenology is perhaps most simply understood as a concern for the client's own subjective meanings. For example, two different clients may present with the same issue or condition, but their own unique interpretation of how that issue or condition might be impacting their lives is likely to be very different. Phenomenological thinking therefore provides the reflexology practitioner with a philosophical framework in which to consider the unique individual experience.

"Phenomenology is vital in ensuring that the client feels understood. (LeBon, 2001)

One of the main problems associated with the increasing clinicalisation of reflexology is personal meaning has the tendency to get somewhat lost under the weight and structure of a medical definition. It is vitally important within any holistic form of therapy not to miss the essential *wholeness* and *variety* of human existence. The practitioner who chooses to consider the inclusion of reflexology as defined alone by a medical definition can often overlook the fuller impact of the individual's experience. The tinnitus client, for example, is affected not only by ringing in the ears, but by emotional distress, a lack of concentration, insomnia, and even fear. The condition can slowly seep into every part of the individual's life, and so to empathically acknowledge and explore this reality; to contextualise it, and help the client to define what they hope to gain from supportive reflexology, is to step into the unique, subjective, phenomenological reality of that particular individual.

Reductionism vs. Holism

The reductionism/holism debate raises questions about the very nature of *"explanation"* itself (McLeod, 2008). For the reductionist to explain a complex phenomenon (like human experience) the phenomenon must be reduced to its constituent parts, whilst the holist considers the whole to be *more* that the sum of the parts.

Reductionism: Noun

- *The practice of analysing and describing a complex phenomenon in terms of its simple of fundamental constituents, especially when this is said to provide a sufficient explanation.*

Holism: Noun

Philosophy:

- *The theory that parts of the whole are in intimate interconnection, such that they cannot exist independently of the whole, or cannot be understood without reference to the whole, which is thus regarded as greater than the sum of its parts.*

Medicine:

- *The treating of the whole person, taking into account mental and social factors, rather than just the symptom of the disease.*

In the counselling and psychotherapy world certainly, most theoretical models (behavioural and psychodynamic) follow a reductionist model, as does the field of medicine in general. The *only* model to adopt a holist viewpoint is **humanism.** Humanism defines an approach which studies the whole person, and the uniqueness of each individual's experience. Humanistic approaches are less interested in *viewing* the experience of a person, but more focused upon trying to understand *through the eyes of the person* having the experience. Therefore the key elements in humanistic thinking are:

- All individuals have free will (within the limitations of their existence).

- Not all behaviours are determined.

- All individuals are born with an innate drive to reach their full potential (self actualisation).

- A fuller understanding of man can only be achieved through studying humans.

- Humanistic studies should consider the individual case (idographic) rather than the average collective performance (nomothetic).

Humanistic thinking is probably most closely associated with Abraham Maslow (1943) - Maslow's Hierarchy of Needs, and Carl Rogers (1951) - Person-Centred Theory.

Existentialism

"A collection of doctrines connected, at bottom, to the view that human beings create meaning in their lives by living, by choosing to exist in a certain way." (Loewer, 2009)

Existentialism is perhaps most associated with the famous French philosopher Jean-Paul Sartre. Sartre proposed the concept of *'bad faith'* or *'mauvaise foi'*, to refer to the strategies employed by individuals to deny freedoms inevitably theirs. In essence, existentialism suggests one cannot escape ones awareness of freedom, simply because it is built into our very consciousness. As such, one might choose to behave in a certain manner – say you eat one cake too many – and then go on to develop a strategy to defend why it wasn't really in you power to stop yourself – when deep inside you really know the power to say no was all yours! Sartre therefore believed the paradox of bad faith is being simultaneously aware and not aware we are free.

Existentialism, Humanism and *Phenomenology* clearly share some important common themes. They each respect the uniqueness of the whole human experience, and value the concept of free choice within that experience.

Limitations in Existentialism, Humanism and Phenomenology

These are certainly also limitations associated with these philosophical and psychological theories:

- They ignore biology and genetics.
- Subjective, therefore considered unscientific (not objective).
- They ignore the sub-conscious mind.
- Difficult to collect qualitative data.

- The belief in free will is in opposition to the deterministic laws of science.

Is it important to consider philosophy in reflexology?

I believe this particular question will answered on an individual practitioner basis. If you consider the power of reflexology lies principally in mechanical manipulation alone then you will probably be fairly uninterested in philosophical thinking. On the other hand, if you consider reflexology to be impacting on a more complex multi-dimensional basis then the concept is more likely to be of interest to you, not just in helping to more clearly define your own professional rationale for practice, but also as a useful therapeutic intervention (mindfulness philosophy, Pooh philosophy, TCM philosophy, etc). Philosophical conversations help to draw out detail and to provide unique context.

- Philosophical thinking can help to provide a framework in which to consider the unique individual experience. In turn this can help to strengthen the quality of the therapeutic relationship, and to promote the concept of autonomy and self directed client change.

- Philosophical thinking can help practitioners to contextualise and formulate more appropriate research studies.

Summary

For too long perhaps the art of reflexology has been considered only from within a rather restrictive *reductionist* framework. This very medical type point of view is unfortunately incapable of incorporating individual perception or personal meaning into any quantifying measurement.

Whilst reflexology is absolutely requiring of this type of scientific and clinical information and measurement, we should perhaps try to consider such quantifiable facts as the *foundations* upon which the more rounded multi-dimensional phenomenological reflexology encounter is seated.

Meeting Stress, Anxiety, Panic and Depression in Reflexology

"When I look back on all these worries, I remember the story of the old man who said on his deathbed that he had a lot of trouble in his life, most of which had never happened."

- Winston Churchill

Stress

Stress is not an illness, but left unmanaged can certainly contribute to the development of more serious illness. Both anxiety and depression can be triggered by stress, as can a host of other more physiologically based disorders.

"Stress is a "complicated cascade of physical and biochemical responses to powerful emotional stimuli." (Mate, 2003)

The experience of stress consists of three components.

1. The physical or emotional (real or perceived) event interpreted as threatening to the individual *(the stress stimulus)*.

2. The processing system responsible for interpreting experience and meaning *(the brain)*.

3. The stress response itself, consisting of both psychological and behavioural reactions and adjustments.

"Stress is fundamentally a response to contextual change. Context is conceptualised in terms of social factors, the influence of other life forms, the non-living aspects of the environment and the characteristics of the individual. (Daruna, 2012)

There are many reasons clients can experience feelings of stress, and it is important to remember the manner in which an individual will react to stressor events is entirely unique.

Common Stress Triggers

Conflict at home or work: Difficult relationship dynamics with spouses, children, and even conflicts arising from responsibilities associated with providing care for elderly relatives can all cause major stress. Additionally, many clients find their workplace to be the major cause of stress in their lives. More and more individuals are working at home on laptops late into the night, as well as having to deal with sometimes complicated relationship dynamics within the workplace.

Major life changes: Divorce, a change of job, a new baby, a house move, redundancy and even retirement can cause stress. Dealing with change can be very difficult for some people. Often individuals can find stress becomes an issue when more than one major life change occurs at the same time.

Lack of time: Family, work and practical home based commitments (cleaning/shopping) can result in some individuals being left with very little free time, and some clients may have been living this way for a considerable length of time.

Negative automatic thinking: Some individuals find life to be stressful and overwhelming simply because they have the tendency to view their experience and the world around them negatively.

Everyone else comes first: Many clients can really benefit from learning that there is a real difference between selfishness and showing oneself some well deserved self-love. Many people spend all their time looking after, and doing for others, and not nearly enough time looking after themselves.

Inability to relax/lack of relaxation: Learning to just 'be' and relax is a real skill. Often individuals require guidance as they learn to relax, and find some peace with their inner thoughts. One reason many people keep themselves so busy is because they can find it difficult to deal with the onslaught of thoughts and feeling that can emerge if they stop dashing around for more than a few minutes.

Unhealthy living: Additive heavy foodstuff, too much alcohol, and a lack of exercise can all compound feelings of stress.

Reflexology and Stress

Encouragingly, increasing numbers of individuals are opting to include therapies such as supportive reflexology within their own personal stress management programmes, and perhaps indeed preventative medicine is the wisest medicine of all. Supportive reflexology can certainly play a positive role in stress management. Reflexology is the only therapy where one is offered the benefit of therapeutic touch and pressure, in addition to an environment in which to develop further life enhancing skills.

Anxiety

Anxiety is the feeling of fear. Anxiety originates from the body's autonomic response to any perceived threat or challenge. Under normal conditions anxiety is not a particularly bad thing. Anxiety can certainly help to motivate us into action when required, and therefore helps to keep us safe. However, when feelings of anxiety begin to spill into other more everyday aspects of life, then the individual may be experiencing a more generalised anxiety disorder.

Physiological Symptoms of Anxiety

- Tense muscles, aches and strains
- Insomnia
- Lethargy

- Stomach and digestive disorders
- Lack of focus and concentration
- Fearing loss of control or rejection
- Feelings of dread, irritability or agitation
- Inability to relax or to control rational thoughts

Reflexology and Anxious Clients

There is a close association between chronic anxiety and the function of the human immune and endocrine systems. High levels of anxiety have also been linked to epi-genetic changes within the body, therefore individuals experiencing inflammatory, endocrine and auto-immune disorders can certainly benefit from supportive reflexology. However, it is important clients who identify anxiety as a potential contributing factor in their health are provided with a new health education philosophy in which to better contextualise their wider health condition and associated general thought processes.

The desire for *certainly* in one's life is perhaps one of the key drivers of anxiety. In order to overcome this stance many clients can benefit from an introduction to mindfulness philosophy and its associated practices. This particular client group can gain tremendously from engaging with a confident, well educated reflexologist.

Panic Attacks

Panic attacks are not dangerous, even though many individuals fear they may be having a heart attack. Panic attacks are defined as a sudden and unexpected surge of severe anxiety. Attacks are very frightening and distressing for the individual. A typical panic attack might last for between 5-30 minutes before the symptoms begin to subside, however, the lasting emotional impact panic attacks can often linger for many hours and even days afterwards.

Symptoms of Panic Attack

- Nausea
- Shaking, dizziness, flushing, sweating
- Chest pain, rapid heart rate, shallow breathing
- Physical numbness and tingling in the extremities
- Feelings of detachment from the surroundings
- Fear of dying, serious illness and loss of control

Reflexology and Panic Attacks

Panic attacks often manifest after major life events such as bereavement or similar type traumatic events. Additionally, panic attacks can manifest in those individuals experiencing elevated levels of sustained stress and anxiety. Whilst reflexology can certainly play a positive part in promoting the well-being concepts of self care, mindful relaxation, and encourage more instances of physiological and emotional homeostasis, it is highly recommended those clients presenting with panic attack are also referred for GP and counselling or psychotherapy support.

Depression

Depression is a serious mental health condition. It is important to understand depression is not just about being a little sad or unhappy. Depression often manifests as a much stronger feeling of hopelessness or deep sadness, and can last for weeks or sometimes many months. Some instances of depression can be rooted in life changes such as divorce, bereavement or employment issues, and sometimes a combination of events contribute to the condition. Other issues like family history, giving birth, social isolation, or long term chronic illness can factor in depression. Some individuals find they battle several bouts of depression throughout their life.

Symptoms of Depression

- Severe low mood
- Feelings of anxiety, worry, guilt, hopelessness
- Lack of motivation and energy
- Aches and pains
- Insomnia
- Appetite changes
- Lack of self care

Reflexology and Depression

As with the panic attack group, perhaps reflexology is best able to support clients experiencing depression through promoting the important well-being concepts of personal self care, and physiological and emotional relaxation. Whilst certainly practitioners can use the reflexology space to promote mindfulness practice for example, the often complicated underlying psychological (and chemical issues) factors involved in clinical depression mean it is also crucial clients gain a referral for GP and counselling or psychotherapy support.

Summary

Perhaps the most important thing to remember about stress, anxiety and depression is not to make assumptions. There is an unfortunate tendency to characterise anxious individuals, for instance, as slightly shaky, incapable and feeble. On the contrary, some of the most anxious people are some of the most capable. These individuals just skilfully learned how to keep their feelings out of sight.

The Therapeutic Relationship in Reflexology

"In my early professional years I was asking the question: How can I treat, or cure, or change this person? Now I would phrase the question in this way: How can I provide a relationship this person may use for his own personal growth."

- Carl Rogers

There are probably only a handful of professional reflexologists unfamiliar with the presence of client emotion in the therapy room. Sometimes clients choose to utilise reflexology hoping to promote a deeper sense of calm and relaxation, perhaps sub-consciously attempting to soothe their inner distress? In other cases emotional content can present alongside an associated physiological issue such as pain, chronic illness, physical exhaustion, or even issues such as sub-fertility.

"Emotional reactions to a series of treatments are not uncommon in bodywork, and the nurturing use of touch and support and acceptance that evolve in the therapeutic relationship may tacitly give permission for this." (Tiran & Mackereth, 2011)

Emotionally Vulnerable Clients

- The phone rings and a potential new client wishes to enquire if you might be able to help him with some night cramps he has been experiencing? He thought having his feet worked on might help with circulation?

- The phone rings and a potential new client wishes to enquire if you might be able to help her with Irritable Bowel Syndrome? The GP suggested she should do things to help her relax?

- The phone rings and a potential new client wishes to enquire if she can book in for reflexology to help her through her upcoming IVF. She read on the internet that reflexology has helped others and she thought relaxation might help?

On the surface it might appear from these examples only the IVF client might require addition consideration in terms of emotional vulnerability. In reality, any one of these example clients might be emotionally vulnerable. It is worth remembering, perhaps not unsurprisingly, that many clients experiencing stress or anxiety related physical disorders can often also feel emotionally stressed, and fairly often will disclose to their reflexology practitioner why that might be.

"Touch has the potential to trigger a catharsis, to be a catalyst for meaningful change, to provide a corrective emotional experience." (Williams et al., 2011)

Undoubtedly, client disclosure, and the presence of emotional content is common place within many reflexology exchanges, and practitioners can choose to deal with the presence of client emotion content in various ways. Some may opt to encourage a more non-verbal, ambiance based setting for their clients, whilst another group may feel more drawn to offer clients a therapeutic safe space in which to share frustrations, fears and worries. Undoubtedly, within every reflexology exchange some form of therapeutic relationship is developing.

Certainly also, it is entirely possible for professional practitioners to consciously engage in a deeper form of therapeutic relationship.

Building Effective Therapeutic Relationships

Person-centred treatment focuses on listening to clients and involving them at a profound level in their own healing, and that requires of the practitioner good communications skills, as well as a technical proficiency in delivering the modality. The term therapeutic relationship is often used to describe the working relationship between any health-care professional, and a client or patient. There are three relating skills, or *ways of being* required to form good effective therapeutic relationships, and they are generally referred to as the *core conditions* (1951).

The Core Conditions

Empathy: *the ability to stand in another person's frame of reference, without losing sight of your own: the ability to try and understand what a client might be feeling or experiencing. Empathy is not the same as sympathy.*

"Empathy fuels connection. Sympathy drives disconnection." - Dr Brene Brown

Empathy is about feeling *with* people. Empathy differs from sympathy. Sympathy is often offered from a metaphorical place of distance; from outside of the individuals experience. Empathy on the other hand, is concerned with stepping into another person's experience, or walking alongside the person in their world. Empathy is therefore also related to reflectively acknowledging the unique experiences and feelings of the individual. The presence of empathy certainly cannot change the client's experience, but empathy can, even for a short time, transform the individuals experience into something less isolating. Empathy also invites us to remain conscious of remembering that as each individual's life experience remains entirely unique, one should never presume to believe they fully understand the individual. In turn, this attitude can help to ensure practitioners are less likely of unwittingly holding *power* within the therapeutic relationship. Empathy reminds us to remain ever mindful of our client's needs - and place value on their right to autonomy, opinion and free choice.

Unconditional Positive Regard: *The client feels valued and accepted as they are: the practitioner may not approve of the client's actions, but the practitioner does wholly approve of the client.*

What does it mean to unconditionally regard a person? It is a big ask really - a huge commitment. To find unconditional acceptance for every client certainly isn't always easy. Ideally though, UPR develops as a part of a practitioner's life philosophy, or personal value system. Perhaps it is best summed up as a way of finding respect for the value of every human being. UPR requires us to find genuine warmth and acceptance for all our clients - indeed all human beings.

No matter how good a person we might *think* we are, or how charitable we might try to be, every individual is judgemental to some degree. Connecting past our judgements to the innate worth and value of each individual is to develop unconditional positive regard. A more non-judgemental attitude can also help to prevent blocks from forming within the therapeutic relationship. It can be easy to disagree with the life choices of a individual, but that disapproval must not be allowed to hinder the fostering of genuine warmth and care within the relationship.

Nourishing the concept of UPR helps us to better demonstrate that our clients are wholly valued and accepted within the relationship just as they are.

Congruence: *genuineness, authentic, being 'real' in the relationship*

This is often the most difficult core condition to define. What does it mean to be *real*? To be real or congruent within the therapeutic relationship might be defined as an attempt to be fully present and aware within each moment, of our own motivations, thoughts and feelings. Human beings have the tendency to demonstrate certain sides of their personalities within many inter-personal exchanges; a certain 'face' for the workplace, another at the hairdresser, and perhaps yet another at home. Practitioners who choose to interact more congruently still retain a professional attitude, but somehow they wish to be experienced as more '*real*' in the manner in which they relate.

The congruent practitioner can be authentic in their interactions, perhaps even braver, for they are truly aware of their inner motivations, ethics and drives. The more congruent practitioner would also avoid taking the role of *authority* figure within the relationship, preferring instead to encourage a more genuine, autonomy promoting exchange; thus respectful of the humanistic concept stating the client remains the *only* true expert in their life and experiencing.

The Collective 'Ways of Being'

Clearly it is difficult to try and connect with any one of the core conditions, without automatically feeling drawn to the remaining two. For true **empathy** to evolve, we must strive to remain **non-judgemental**, and for that to occur we find we are propelled towards becoming more **congruent** with, and attentive to, our own personal thoughts, opinions and experiencing.

In essence it is the 'blending' of these three relating skills which defines the nature and quality of the therapeutic relationship.

Ideally, the *'ways of being'* come to develop as natural extension of the practitioners true self; as the practitioner become more real, so too can every relationship and interaction. A more natural ability to demonstrate the core conditions often flourishes in line with the depth of self development and awareness a practitioner holds. The core conditions might essentially be perceived as human skills, finely tuned and intensified during focused therapeutic exchanges.

The practitioner *use of self* within the therapeutic relationship might be likened to the sum total of the core conditions, blended and demonstrated to the client through the personality and uniqueness of the practitioner. There is no mask of authority to be worn in the consulting room. Rather, there exists a genuine human presentation of clarity of thought and focus, fully engaged in the world of another. It is simply one human being genuinely and non-judgmentally meeting another in their world, offering a caring, supportive ear.

Summary

Our innately multi-dimensional modality offers not only a powerful touch and pressure therapy, but also an intimate face to face encounter; a perfect therapeutic combination, and one perhaps unique to the reflexology package. Conscious therapeutic relationships not only provide our more emotionally vulnerable clients with a safe and supportive space for disclosure, and the sharing of emotional content, but the relationship can also provide an interaction capable of promoting appropriate client education, and increased levels of autonomy.

Effective therapeutic relationships keep clients safe, they allow professional practitioners to engage with clients in a deeper, perhaps more meaningful ways, and finally, they hold the potential to re-ignite a client's drive towards more self acceptance, and better levels of self care.

As a valuable CAM profession, as we begin to learn more about the therapeutic relationship, something I am confident many practitioners are providing quite instinctively, we are also beginning to champion its very real existence, and therapeutic value, within the complex multi-dimensional reflexology package.

Practitioner Self Development

"As human beings, our greatness lies not so much in being able to remake the world - that is the myth of the atomic age - as in being able to remake ourselves."

- Mahatma Gandhi

The concept of self development (or self-awareness) should be important to any individual engaging with individuals therapeutically. High levels of self-awareness can provide the practitioner with a better understanding of their own drives, motivations, feelings, moods, and strengths. More self-aware individuals tend to experience deeper levels of self acceptance, and are often better able to experience themselves within all relationships more authentically and congruently. Additionally, deeper levels of self awareness can help to refine our thoughts and opinions and to identify what really makes us happy. Often increased self-awareness empowers the individual to make changes in their life and to self actualising - to become all they can be. Knowing oneself more intimately can make it easier to identify and refine what is really important. Self-awareness therefore can help the individual to ditch the unwanted, and to travel lighter through life.

Within a professional therapeutic context practitioner self awareness is vitally important - principally because without it therapeutic relationships are often more difficult to build, and to maintain. A lack of sufficient practitioner self awareness can result in power heavy relationships, judgmental verbal reflections, and even a general lack of meaningful empathy. Additionally high levels of self-awareness can help to reduce the possibility of transference/counter-transference occurring within therapeutic relationships. Therefore, self-awareness also helps to ensure active promotion of client autonomy and self directed change.

Another good and valid justification for engaging in adequate self development relates to the concept of *respect*, and working ethically with those more emotionally vulnerable groups. Good levels of self awareness can help practitioners to develop effective professional boundaries, and to recognise more quickly when a professional referral may be required.

Respecting the boundaries of our modality, and indeed the limitations of our own professional competencies, helps to ensure practitioners remain mindful of appreciating each client's entirely unique stance, and their very real presenting needs. Thus self-awareness also helps to ensure we continue to work professionally and ethically.

Finally, self development is heavily linked to the concept of practitioner self-care, and therefore also the avoidance of practitioner burnout. Self care within this particular context really means to treat ourselves with the same level of care and respect we try to demonstrate to our clients. Practitioners can undoubtedly take steps towards avoiding losing touch with their own personal power, through engaging in adequate levels of self care, and potentially even instances of professional supervision.

Self development is an integral part of developing wider therapeutic skills. Personal awareness can really only be truly measured by the individual. How much are you worth investing in, and how does the concept of self development relate to your own personal and professional rationale for practice?

Professional Supervision

One clear benefit related to working as a reflexologist within a multi-disciplinary environment is undoubtedly the provision of profession supervision. Many practitioners starting out in practice, as well as those engaging with more emotionally vulnerable client groups might also benefit from the provision of more structured professional support. How best to introduce the concept of professional supervision in reflexology presents our industry with another weighty future challenge. Supervision is not about teaching as such, but more about support and mentoring and even offering other perspectives.

Looking past the more basics aspects of professional support, (which currently many practitioners access via local and online peer support), an experienced supervisor can also help the practitioner with other, more complex issues. These issues might involve a difficult relational dynamic with a particular client perhaps, or feelings of overwhelming responsibility. In such cases supervision can be a useful place to work through any feelings of transference or counter-transference, and to redefine professional boundaries. This form of support can also be invaluable in terms encouraging and developing practitioner self awareness, particularly when the practitioner is able to build up a more long term relationship with their supervisor.

Group Supervision

Over and above developing mentoring opportunities within the industry (experienced practitioners more formally supervising less experienced) perhaps one of the most useful ways to introduce the concept of supervision would be for small groups of practitioners to join forces and invite along a local supervisor on a monthly/bimonthly basis. Ideally any supervisor would hold duel training (reflexology/counselling), or a counsellor possessing a good appreciation of the reflexology relationship. Those readers retaining membership with modality organisations offering local groups support, might raise this suggestion with their fellow group members.

"Apart from using group time for discussion, they might consider devising experiential exercises or introducing role playing techniques. The who point is they should find colleagues to share new learning opportunities, address difficulties or other problems together, and pay heed to warning when outburst is spotted by fellow carers, and, - most importantly - to take heart from encouragement." (March-Smith, 2005)

Working in isolation can be challenging. Our industry presently under values the concept of professional supervision unfortunately. As we move forward in presenting some of the complexities involved in our modality, so too it might be useful to start to honour some of the complexities practitioners are dealing with on a daily basis, and begin to construct a professional network capable of appropriately supporting the professional development and emotional health of professional reflexology practitioners.

Note: Each of us ultimately holds personal responsibility for keeping oneself safe. If you become aware of any emotional content surfacing as you read through any of the articles, it is highly recommended that you find a safe way to work through that content, either by engaging with a local supportive counsellor, or by accessing supportive peer contact.

Winnie the Pooh Psychology
A Reflective Practitioner Exercise

"Think it over, think it under."

- Winnie the Pooh

This article has been constructed principally as a practitioner self development tool. In some instances it may also be appropriate to utilise the tool with clients. There are several important points to consider should a practitioner feel drawn towards sharing this information with clients, and those topics are covered in the final section of the article. Let us now turn our attention to the inhabitants of the Hundred Acre Wood.

Pooh Bear

In the field of **humanistic** psychology the concept of **self actualisation** is an important one. The self actualising individual has clearly identified who they really are, and what brings them real happiness and fulfillment.

"Sometimes,' said Pooh, 'the smallest things take up the most room in your heart."

This individual is reaching their own unique potential, within the limitations of their environment. This self-actualising individual is considered therefore to be both self-aware and self-determining, and able to live each day consciously connected to their present experiencing.

"For I am a bear of very little brain."

Pooh is really a very smart little bear, despite what he might have you believe. Pooh certainly seems to have identified what makes him truly happy, and that of course is honey! Pooh is self actualising every day, becoming all he can be, and doesn't care too much about what others *think* he should become. Pooh also tries very hard not to fill his brain with too many troublesome worries, preferring instead to adopt a more mindful approach to his thinking. Big words Pooh finds simply exhausting! Granted, outside of the Hundred Acre Wood, perhaps Pooh's work attendance record might not be too impressive, after all, with honey to cause such distraction it might well prove difficult for Pooh to go to work *every* single weekday! However, in terms of living as a self-directed and actualised individual, knowing what really makes his heart sing, Pooh certainly seems to have it mastered.

Pooh says he is entirely happy to stay for lots of reflexology, just so long as he can bring his honey too?

Eeyore

Eeyore can be a bit of a challenge for the inhabitants of the Hundred Acre Wood. Some have even suggested Eeyore is clinically depressed. Eeyore's glass certainly seems to be half empty, and much in his world seems to be an enormous struggle. He really is rather gloomy.

"End of the road. Nothing to do, and no hope of things getting better."

Eeyore can though help us to identify and honour our feelings of sadness and tiredness. Sometimes it is only through allowing ourselves to genuinely connect to our real feelings of exhaustion that we can start the process of releasing our associated physiological stress. Trauma, sadness and stress can linger deep in our cells and tissues and Eeyore teaches to be mindful of honouring and expressing our feelings; giving them voice, both verbally *and* through the felt sense. Eeyore also reminds us that whilst it is never a good idea to linger in a negative place for too very long, neither should we feel compelled to pretend to be happy or energetic. Sadness is simply a sometimes unavoidable part of life, just as it is an unavoidable but very real element of the magical Hundred Acre Wood.

Eeyore thinks whatever reflexology is, it doesn't sound like it's for him at all, and even he did have some 'ology he feels it surely wouldn't help him one bit. Oh no, nothing can do that really. Oh well . . .

Piglet

Piglet is full of worries, and thoughts, and concerns, and maybes, and what if's? Piglet's anxiety levels are certainly very high, and his *Hypothalamus-Pituitary-Adrenal axis* is likely to be on high alert from the very moment he wakes.

"Supposing a tree fell down, Pooh, when we were underneath it?' 'Supposing it didn't,' said Pooh after careful thought. Piglet was comforted by this."

Piglet worries over just about everything and everyone in the Hundred Acre Wood, even making sure to find time to worry about the things he hasn't even considered worrying about yet. It is all very tiring really, all this living in the future and so mostly, Piglet prefers to stay at home where it feels much safer. Piglet of course has his positive traits too. He reminds us to stay safe. We can all benefit from a healthy dose of Piglets ability to ponder and consider more fully. Piglets thinking, in balanced good measure, can help us to make more informed decisions, and even help us to fine tune our intuition and inner guiding voice. Piglet can help us to stop and wait a while, pondering a little deeper, before we dive in fully.

Piglet would like to know, if it's not too much trouble, if reflexology will be uncomfortable and he would also like to know if you are familiar with working on such little toes? They are his only toes and he is really very fond of them. Perhaps it's not a very good idea? He thinks your hands look rather large. What if it tickles? Oh dear – he's not so very sure now?

Rabbit

Some of the animals in the Hundred Acre Wood think Rabbit is a bit of a control freak. Rabbit has very strong opinions (on just about everything) and he certainly isn't shy about sharing them, nor is he shy about hammering up the odd sign or two informing the other animals on how to behave. In his own way attempting to direct the chaos he sees all around.

"Owl," said Rabbit shortly, "you and I have brains. The others have fluff. If there is any thinking to be done in this forest – and when I say thinking I mean thinking – you and I must do it."

Rabbit's heightened sense of right and wrong is never more challenged than when someone walks across his perfectly tended to vegetable patch. Rabbit really does find the other animals quite infuriating sometimes. Rabbit's positivity lies perhaps in his organisational skills and in his sense of pride. Rabbit wholeheartedly believes a job should be done to the best of one's ability, and Rabbit always plans his time and day well. He tries never to waste a moment.

Rabbit would like the reflexology to commence at exactly 2pm because he has carrots to plant later. Rabbit would also like to know how long exactly you have been trained in Reflexology, can he see your qualifications, and have you ever worked with rabbit feet before? Rabbit would also prefer to rotate his own ankles during the session, thank you very much.

Tigger

Rarely sad or tired like his friend Eyore, Tigger seems to bounce happily through life and his various adventures. Tigger certainly doesn't pause as Piglet might to consider possible dangers, nor does Tigger plan ahead as Rabbit might. Tigger prefers instead to bounce off into new adventures without much of an idea of what he might encounter. Tigger's you see, apparently *never* get lost!

"Bouncy, trouncy, flouncy, pouncy, fun, fun, fun, fun, fun. The most wonderful thing about Tigger's is I'm the only one!"

Tigger's positivity does not lie in his careless attitude, but rather in his *carefree* attitude. It could be argued that Tigger remains firmly and healthily attached to his own inner child, his sense of freedom, his sense of fun and his seemingly boundless levels of enthusiasm and energy. Being a grown up is entirely too serious sometimes, and we can all learn a little from Tigger's love of bouncing and adventure.

"I'm so happy I could bounce."

Tigger says he thinks reflexology is just FANTASTIC and wants to know if you can rub his other paws too, because being a Tigger he has four feet, don't you know?

Summary

Perhaps then we each require just a little of each of our furry friends characteristics. Problems tend to occur when we find we are leaning too far into one set of behaviours or patterns. Pooh can help us to stay connected to who we really are, and to identify what is important to us. He reminds us to strive for self actualisation in our lives, and about the importance of demonstrating kindness, to both ourselves and to others.

Eeyore helps us to honour our emotions, including our sadness and feelings of isolation or stress. Through Eeyore we can also help to heal the physical body, and find worth in releasing some of our long held pain and hurt. Eeyore reminds us to listen to our felt sense and to honour our heart.

Piglet reminds us to stay safe and to make more considered and thought out decisions, helping to keep us safe. Piglet also reminds us not to allow fear to overwhelm us or to decide our path. Rabbit can help us to organise our life, and take pride in our actions. He offers structure, patience and faith. He also reminds us of the determination, and sometimes arrogance of the ego. Rabbit therefore also reminds us to be humble.

Finally, Tigger can help us to remain connected to the spontaneity of life. He reminds us to laugh, to have fun and to be kind and welcoming to all we encounter. Most importantly, Tigger reminds us to embrace our life.

As a Practitioner Self Development Tool

The idea of the exercise is to try and support the practitioner as they identify personal similarities with one (or two) of the characters described, or perhaps the practitioner might experience benefit from adopting the characteristics of yet another?

- Have you identified what really makes you happy in your life? What is your honey? Are there some areas of your life you feel are more complete and satisfying? Are there other things to be worked on? Added to? Developed? Perhaps instead you spend too little time with your *honey* - finding you struggle to manage the demands of life or expectation? Can you find a more balanced place? What else might make you happy?

- Are you as mindful with your thoughts as Pooh seems to be, or does your mind race more like Piglet's? If you are a piglet type thinker can you identify why that might be? Did you learn the behaviour from another, or did an event occur perhaps to make you wary in life? Do you tend to catastrophize events and blow them out of proportion? Or perhaps feelings of fear and anxiety limit your life? Does Piglets anxiety restrict your own behaviour?

- Perhaps you are more familiar with Rabbit's daily frustration, or maybe you require a little more of Rabbit's organisational skills and determination? Do you feel frustrated with the world, and its inhabitants? Do you have some of your own signs you'd like to knock up?

- Perhaps you feel you could do with a dose of Tigger's carefree attitude? Have you been stuck in the grind too long? When did you last have a good belly laugh, or spontaneous adventure? Do you love *you* enough? Are you paying enough attention to the here and now?

Now try to think about how these possible characteristics and trends might be affecting you as a therapist?

- How do you feel for example about the client who consistently seems to be melancholily, or lacking in any motivation to change? Do you ever feel frustrated by this type of client? Perhaps you feel sad during, or after working with this type of client? Have you perhaps encountered the client who presents exhausted by responsibility having forgotten there are other things in life capable of drawing a smile? Does it take more from you to work with the melancholy client?

- How do you manage the anxious client who seems to require constant guidance and re-assurance? Do you find this to be endearing, draining or perhaps even irritating? How do feel about the two steps forward, one backwards journey that often accompanies the anxious client? What happens when this type of client calls you at 9pm looking for assurance, or wants to meet for a friendly coffee? How about the anxious client cancelling appointments at the last minute, always experiencing one emergency or another?

- How do you feel about the tetchy client with an answer for everything and an often argumentative tone? Does it feel like a power struggle sometimes? Do clients like these make you feel intimidated, or more determined to have your say? Might you be a bossy Rabbit type practitioner who always knows best, if so, what happens when you meet another rabbit? That might not be a long relationship?

A Healthy Blend

It is important to remember there is no right or wrong answer to any of the example questions. The purpose of the exercise is to encourage you to think more about how you relate with certain individuals and different personality types. We each ideally hold a combination of the characters traits. The real question is how balanced are these traits, in your personality, and with your clients? Good therapeutic relationships are constructed on the foundations of empathy, congruence and unconditional positive regard. It can be helpful to become better acquainted with our own inner narrative and practitioner opinions if we wish to engage on a deeper relational level, or to hope to encourage client autonomy. What happens for example when a Piglet practitioner meets an Eeyore client? Should the timid Piglet practitioner eventually challenge the pessimistic, self sabotaging Eeyore type client? Is it ok to continue to take money from a client seemingly gaining nothing from the encounter? Or perhaps the Eeyore client meets a rabbit type practitioner? How much patience might Rabbit have with Eeyore's lack of pro-activeness? Or perhaps the piglet practitioner meets the bossy rabbit client - intimidating perhaps? How do you really feel as a therapist when a client starts ever sentence with 'yes, but ...'? Frustrated? Irritated? Useless? Inadequate?

Engaging in self development can help us to become more actively aware of our own inner judgments and opinions. In turn, this can help to prevent blocks from forming within therapeutic relationships. Play with the ideas. Try to think about how you view yourself in relation to other people within your own personal circle. Do you have a timid voice, or a loud voice? How do you feel about authority and being told what to do? Annoyed or comforted? Try to get to know yourself even better. You might choose to consider thinking about:

- **Family** relationships and **Friendships**

- Relationships with real or perceived **authority** figures. How do you feel about rules and regulations, or those individuals with very fixed opinions? Do you like being told what to do? Are you a leader, or a follower? Do you perhaps feel safer with very assertive people, or do they make you silently quiver?

- Relationships with those of a different **age** group, **sexual** orientation, **ethnic** background, or **culture**. Do you find you become more submissive when dealing with older people for example?

- Your relationship with **yourself**. What annoys you about you? What do you love and value about you? What are your qualities, and might there be something involving you requires more attention?

As a Reflective Tool with Clients

This reflective tool is born from experiences in my own therapy room. I have used the concept to both help clients identify how they might be feeling, and often to help clients focus on what is really important in their life. The concept is relatively simple with three of the characters (*Eeyore, Piglet and Rabbit*) representing the most commonly encountered personality sub-types presenting for reflexology. There are a few important issues to consider before deciding to share this information with clients:

- The tool is **not** relevant for every reflexology client and should only be used within an existing therapeutic relationship where the practitioner and the client feel comfortable in each other's company. This is **not** a first session tool.

- The tool can be particularly helpful in those instances where the practitioner becomes aware of clients repetitive patterns. For example, the client who often fails to make beneficial dietary changes will often identify with either Eeyore or Piglet. Whilst the client who tells you she is too busy to find time for self care will often feel more to drawn to Rabbit.

- NEVER try to guide a client based on your opinion. Rather present the story in a *lighthearted* manner, and trust your client will find themselves drawn to the appropriate characters.

Based on new information clients can start to think about how to invoke change, i.e., more self care, less worry, more assertiveness, and so on. Lighthearted philosophical conversations can help the client to define a helpful path forward.

Relational Reflexology

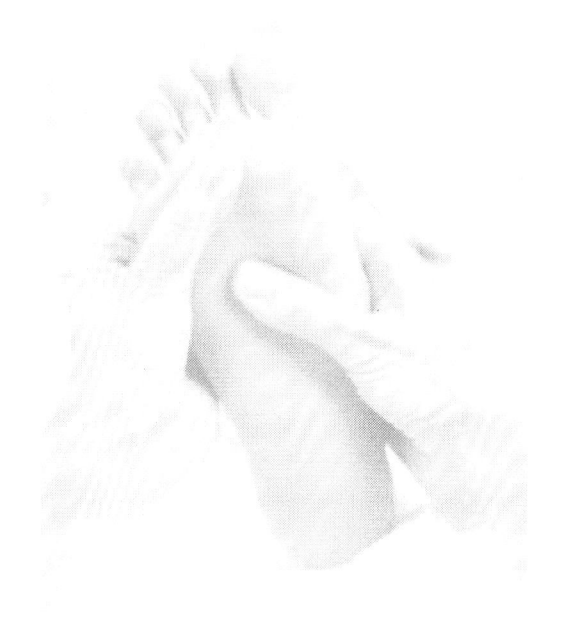

Power and Responsibility in the Reflexology Relationship

"The measure of a man is what he does with power."

– Plato

Power is an element occurring in many everyday human relationships. Consider for a moment the relationship between a parent and child, a teacher and pupil, a manager and worker, a doctor and patient? In many commonly experienced every day human relationships power is certainly present. In some cases power can provide a useful element of social or employment structure. Sometimes power is cultural in origin.

Does Power Exist in Reflexology?

Elements of power exist in all therapeutic relationships. Most typically power issues manifest as sub-conscious forms of transference and counter-transference. Sometimes power can present more explicitly, for example through associations with titles, uniforms and even environment. Consider for a moment the manner in which a client might perceive the professional reflexology practitioner working from within a hospital or clinical setting? How might this relationship differ from one formed with a home based practitioner? Might the client view the hospital based practitioner more formally, simply because of environment, or even because of practitioner attire? Now take some time to consider how much power a practitioner is given to hold when engaging with an emotionally vulnerable and physically exhausted client; one so tired they almost seem to fall unreservedly into your safe care and hands?

Certainly different forms of power have the potential to manifest within therapeutic relationships, and they can often be tied up with the concept of responsibility.

Understanding Transference and Counter-Transference

Transference literally means to *'carry across'* (Fox, 2008), and was a phrase first coined by the psychodynamic theorist, Sigmund Freud, to label the way he felt patients transferred feelings about, and stemming from, important people in their early lives, onto their therapist. Counter-transference relates directly to the feelings the therapist develops towards the patient.

"Understanding transference and counter-transference can be useful in the therapeutic alliance. It can open up a whole new dimension to the healing environment, if only in the benign guise of child and parent together." (March-Smith, 2005)

Perhaps the most important aspect relating to the concept of transference occurring within a reflexology context relates to the possibility of accepting, or adopting, a position of power within the relationship. Power can be given to the practitioner, and the practitioner can also choose to hold power.

"Every practitioner knows that the patient has walked into the consulting room in the hope they will be made to feel better." (March-Smith, 2005)

Rosie March-Smith's statement (above) highlights the potential weight of responsibility often silently placed upon the professional reflexology practitioners shoulders. Many of our clients attend for reflexology because of chronic illness, pain, or exhaustion. Every day professional practitioners are asked to take on the responsibility of trying to help clients feel better.

Transference in Action

In some cases a clients need to be cared for might be sub-consciously transferred onto the practitioner. Perhaps in this case the client is transferring a deep inner need for touch, attention and care, at the same time becoming almost childlike in their passiveness towards better health.

- In unwittingly giving power away is this client inhibiting their potential towards increased self-care?

- How might such a relationship impact the practitioner?

- Might the practitioner feel empowered?

- Tired? Overwhelmed?

- What does the felt sense say?

Another example might be the client who seems quite determined to retain their condition and experience; repeatedly reporting no change, yet still insist on attending for sessions. Perhaps this client is transferring their own need to retain some form of authority, whilst still gaining from the encounter in some manner?

- Why do clients such as these continue to attend?

- What feelings can clients such as these present to the practitioner?

- Responsibility? Fear? Helplessness? Pressure? Needing to apologise?

- What does the felt sense say?

Perhaps in another example the client fears disappointing the practitioner, worrying they may damage their new found friendship, potentially transferring fears of rejection?

- Is there something identifiable preventing a more authentic relationship?

- Is the practitioner aware of any sense of responsibility?

- Are there feelings of flattery? Pressure?

- What does the felt sense say?

Counter-Transference and the Wounded Healer

"We might replace the words Great Healer with Good Father or Good Mother, understanding that there is a similarity with the role of a caring, attentive parent offering, seemingly, endless time for this needy child: someone to take away the hurt, effectively to 'kiss it better', to murmur reassuring words, and to make the consulting room seem just like a cosy room at home from their childhood." (March-Smith, 2005)

Some theorists have suggested that counter-transference is present in some form at the very onset of many therapeutic encounters. The practitioners own initial sub-conscious call towards engaging in therapeutic work; their inner requirement to nourish and help care for others, representing a reflection of the practitioners own inner child's need for care. Researchers suggest the ability to empathise develops to such an advanced degree in childhood that these adult individuals can often feel compelled to care for others, and feel drawn towards more therapeutic professions.

"The presence of such a 'wound' in a healer gives them an excellent basis from which to understand and empathise with the wounds of clients." (McLoud, 1998)

Practitioner Self Development

Highlighting some of the finer dynamics involved in relational encounters, such as becoming aware of the possibility of transference and counter-transference, and, indeed concepts such as the wounded healer help to demonstrate the real demand for good levels of self awareness in professional reflexology practitioners. Practitioners can certainly benefit from enhanced levels of self development, becoming more swiftly able to recognise instances of transference of counter-transference and able to take steps towards promoting more autonomous exchanges; choosing ultimately not to take responsibility for their clients.

Some of our wider therapeutic reflexology interactions then clearly possess hidden subconscious dynamics; dynamics not only capable of hindering the promotion of client autonomy and free choice, but when left unchecked can also induce practitioner burn out. Practitioners who engage therefore in more regular instances of reflective self development can promote higher standards of client care, and increase their own levels of practitioner self care.

Recognising Somatic Counter-Transference

"We could say that all counter-transference, all the feelings that arise in the practitioner in relation to the client, are somatic counter-transference." (Fox, 2008)

Practitioners might recognise instances of somatic counter-transference in their own felt sense responses. Perhaps the feeling might manifest as an overwhelming sense of tiredness as the practitioner works on the client, or it might display as a feeling of sickness or anxiety? On a different occasion there might be a feeling of irritation or frustration, or perhaps even an awareness of tears emerging? It is worth spending some time examining what the felt sense means to you personally?

Within The Therapeutic Relationship

The concepts of transference and counter-transference are not directly associated with the concept of building therapeutic relationships, but they are certainly worth becoming more familiar with.

"The reality is that transference phenomena belong to a much more superficial level of relating where people are still being symbols for each other." (Means & Cooper, 2005)

Offering our clients the core conditions associated with a therapeutic relationship (empathy, congruence and unconditional positive regard), can help to reduce instances of transference and counter-transference occurring in the relationship. Additionally practitioners are better able to promote the concepts of client autonomy and self-directed change, principally through encouraging more authentic, empathically driven, relational encounters.

We practitioners certainly play an enormous role in invoking some of the changes our client's experience. It is important therefore we become more professionally aware and attentive to our potentially powerful, very real impact.

Other Instances of Power Manifesting in Reflexology

The Association of Reflexologists (UK) posted an interesting question on their public Facebook page recently - a question highlighting perfectly one example of a potential power concept manifesting in reflexology.

- 'Do clinical uniforms actually cause a barrier between client and therapist?'

One of the contributors to the thread, enquired?

- Do clients trust and respect as soon as they see a uniform, and is this a good thing? What is the intention of wearing a uniform?

- Does wearing a uniform give someone power? Does it empower or disempower you or the client? '

If we consider the concept of transference and counter-transference, then what message might we be potentially portraying when we adopt a clinical type uniform?

Are we projecting the belief we can be trusted? Does our uniform say something about our intentions?

- What message are we potentially portraying to our clients, who all too frequently present craving change and autonomy, when we greet them in a clinical type uniform?

- Is it really about keeping clean, or adopting 'professional' attire? What do we mean by professional? Do we mean clinical? Might there be something about feeling we should align reflexology with something more medically and clinically acceptable? Does the uniform make it ok?

- Might there be something in us (the therapist) that feels safer associated with something more clinically acceptable? Does the uniform help to form the persona of the therapist?

Taking time to consider some of these questions more closely can help us to challenge some of our own judgements and assumptions. Can we somehow present professionally wearing non-clinical work attire? How might that be possible? What elements might be required?

Try to remember there are no wrong answers. We are all unique, and our opinions and personal boundaries are varied.

Summary

Thinking a little deeper about how we relate with, and indeed present ourselves to clients, is not only an ethically positive stance to adopt, but such consideration also helps us to relate with clients in a deeper, more meaningful way; without any perceived label of authority.

"Relations between people are the basis of social and individual lives, and relational concepts are used to understand human life in all its complexity." (Paul & Pelham, 2000)

It seems important as a profession we strive to stand in the true light of our modalities complex and innate power to invoke change multi-dimensionally. If we are to further champion specifically the role of the practitioner, for example, then we must also become more accustomed with some of the components most often considered within a therapeutic relating context.

"Being alert to whatever may emerge from the unconscious might seem like extra and unexpected responsibility for the hardworking complementary practitioner. It could however, be a taste of things to come: for, as the government continues to tackle the lack of regulation nationwide, it is likely more and more training bodies will enhance their

curricula to include a working knowledge of concepts such as transference and counter-transference, projection and projective identification. (March-Smith, 2005)

Ultimately good levels of practitioner self development and heightened self awareness help to reduce the possibility of power imbalances, and transference and counter-transference occurring within the therapeutic relationship. Practitioners might find it helpful to discuss these topics further within supportive peer support or local group meetings. Try to more finely define the path to knowing you are enough. That you the practitioner, within the context of the therapeutic relationship and supported by the physical component of the modality, have the capability to invoke therapeutic change.

There is simply no requirement for the concept of power when we try to find genuine concern for another human being.

The Felt Sense, Interpretation and Mindfulness in Reflexology

"Men are not moved by things but by their interpretations."

- Epictetus

The bodily **felt sense** is a significant phenomenon associated with person-centred counselling and body-oriented psychotherapy. It is essentially the observation of one's own sensory and visceral experiences.

Visceral: Adjective

1. Relating to the viscera: the visceral nervous system.

2. Relating to deep inward feelings, rather than intellect.

The felt sense is experienced in the physical body and has been defined as a pre-verbal sense of *'something'*, an inner knowledge or awareness, not yet consciously verbalised. The felt sense can sometimes represent an old wound or hurt, recognition of a present situation, or even a future insight or idea.

The Felt Sense in Counselling

Within a counselling context part of the talking therapist's role is to help the client through means of visualisation, focusing techniques and verbal exchanges, to better access their bodily felt sense, and attempt to bring forth a more defined awareness.

"This experience of discovering within oneself present attitudes and emotions which have been viscerally and physiologically experienced, but have never been

recognised in consciousness, constitutes one of the deepest and most significant phenomena of therapy." (Rogers, 1951)

The Felt Sense in Reflexology

Within a reflexology context it is quite possible a similar phenomenon is occurring quite spontaneously, simply as a result of the rapid focus of attention brought to the client's physical body responses through the medium of touch and pressure.

"The way in which the reflexologist works, offering body reflections in conjunction with reflexology techniques, and the way the counsellor works using contact reflections, constitutes an allocation of the client's attention – primarily to their physical responses to their environment and to treatment, and subsequently to areas of emotional response." (Uphoff, 1999)

In order to better understand this phenomenon, and how it might be manifesting within a reflexology context let us now consider the fairly typical client who attends for reflexology with painful, swollen or stagnated lung or diaphragm reflexes.

The Lung and TCM

The lung essentially supports the heart and circulation. TCM philosophy states lung energy can become depleted as a result of deep stress and over-thinking. Anxiety caused by persistent stress causes deeper injury to the lung energy.

Both shallow and irregular breathing are therefore considered to be a symptom of anxiety. Anxiety can also cause problems in the fu organ associated with the lung – the large intestine (for example, over-anxious individuals can be prone to ulcerative colitis and IBS).

Zang-Fu Organ Associations

- Zang Organ: Lung

- Fu Organ: Large Intestine

- Sensory Organ: Nose/Skin

- Emotions: Anxiety, Grief, Over-thinking (Cognitive Activity), Deep Stress

- Active Time: 3-5 am (Lung) 5-7am (Large intestine)

The Lung and Diaphragm in Reflexology

Chris Stormer (2007) writes about the general reflex area:

"The balls of the feet take on the bulk of the body, as well as some of the more hefty emotions, whilst at the same time, revealing the amount of self esteem that comes from feelings towards one and others."

The diaphragm reflexes (abdominal brain), also situated in the general area, draw's our attention further to a strong connection between intense emotional states and the wider digestive system.

"The solar plexus is a highly emotional part of the body, connected to the element of air, which physically, emotionally and spiritually links the soul to its surroundings. This is why any interaction through the breath or speech, can have such a profound effect on it and the digestive tract." (Stormer, 2007)

The Effect of the Fight or Flight Response

The aim of the fight or flight response is to keep us safe, and it is a vital part of our most basic human survival mechanisms. The mind and fear trigger the fight or flight response, in reaction to whatever the mind experiences as both real and perceived danger.

"Fear and anxiety are our natural states of being, assisting us in our survival. (Collard, 2013)

When danger is perceived, the hypothalamus activates two systems – the sympathetic nervous system and the adrenal-cortical system. The fight or flight response is characterised by:

- The involvement of the sympathetic nervous system ensures the body speeds up, ready to take action. The respiratory and heart rate increases along with blood pressure, whilst signals are sent to the muscles readying them to be alert.

- The stress hormones epinephrine (adrenaline) and norepinephrine (noradrenaline) are released into the bloodstream by the adrenal gland.

- The hypothalamus releases corticotropin-releasing factor (CRF) into the pituitary gland, activating the adrenal-cortical system. The pituitary gland in turn secretes the hormone ACTH (adrenocorticotropic hormone) which moves through the bloodstream, arriving at the adrenal cortex where it activates the release of other hormones that help the body prepare to deal with the threat.

- Non-essential systems like **digestion** are shut down. Blood is redistributed away from the digestive tract and sent instead to the muscles and limbs, thus providing extra energy and fuel.

Impacting Through Interpretation

So now we have collated three individual interpretations (including a clinical definition). Each one clear in suggesting that intense, repetitive, and perhaps even deep seated historical emotions and feelings have the potential to directly impact the lung (respiratory rate) and the digestive system. How might the professional practitioner best utilise this philosophical and clinical information safely with reflexology clients?

Reflection in the Therapy Room

The key to the safe use of interpretation in the reflexology room lies in developing the skill of reflection. A reflection is neither a question or a statement of fact, but rather a simple, clear acknowledgment of what the listener can see, hears, feels, or may be aware of. Let us now consider a possible scenario in which we might come to utilise such reflective responses:

Client: *'That bit feels sore. What is it?'*

Therapist: *'This area represents the lungs in reflexology.'*

Client: *'Does that mean I have something wrong with my lungs?'*

Therapist: *'No, not at all. Sometimes this area displays as sensitive or gritty when an individual is prone to frequent respiratory conditions, and sometimes it can display when a person is dealing with a lot of stress. According to TCM the lungs are linked to over thinking and a busy mind – and also to more historic grief or feelings of sadness.*

Client: *'That sounds a bit like me. I tend to think quite a lot. My mind never seems to slow down.'*

Therapist: *'Ok - According to TCM, when unbalanced, lung energy can wake a person between 3-5am, when the meridian is most active.'*

Client: *'That's me! I often wake at 4am and can't get back to sleep.'*

Therapist: *'Close your eyes for a moment and take a deep breath. Now bring your attention in towards your chest and abdominal area. How does that area feel like to you just now?'*

Client: *'It feels quite tight and ….. heavy.'*

The client's final interpretation of tight and heavy is a direct representation of their own felt sense. This reflective response example demonstrates clearly that the therapist makes no attempt to interpret on behalf of the client, but rather simply offers the information for the clients own consideration. Interacting empathically (from within the clients own frame of reference) and reflectively helps to ensure the therapist does not unwittingly retain power within the therapeutic relationship.

There is no requirement to make any further emotional interpretation, or to attempt to add more detail to what has already been identified or offered by the client. Within a reflexology context it is important not to try and delve too far into a client's emotional background, or to try and unravel a particular psychology, no matter how tempting it may be. Practitioners can certainly choose to expand on any further relevant philosophical or clinical information, but must remain mindful of leaving any interpretation to the client. In a relational reflexology encounter focus should be towards attempting to encourage the client's attention back to their present unique phenomenological experiencing, and any associated bodily felt sense.

Calming The Stormy Mind

In today's modern busy world it has become increasingly common for individuals to become detached from their innate physiological felt sense, and their ability to read the internal signals their body sends. The pressures of modern life, with our determination to do well and achieve and our personal inner drives to find acceptance, and a perfect piece of happiness, have unfortunately resulted in an increasing level of disassociation from our true emotional states.

"The result of a lifestyle that is 100 percent different from how people lived for thousands of years is a lack of peace, lack of enjoyment and a number of destructive emotions that lead to psychosomatic disease." (Collard, 2013)

Clients experiencing long term disappointment, anxiety, sadness and chronic illness, can often develop a deep inner world in which they retreat to dwell, or to further consider their difficult situation. Frustration stemming from feelings of powerlessness, sadness, pain, and even a lack of hope, can lead to further anxiety and negative automatic thinking patterns developing.

"A great deal of our daily brain activity is left-brain activation: thinking, planning, evaluating and so on. It is surprising we are not lopsided considering how much we 'think and therefore feel we are (Descartes, French philosopher) and how little time we spend truly connected to one of our feeling senses in the right brain." (Collard, 2013)

The promotion of any activity capable of encouraging more focused, attentive, relaxation states can therefore prove beneficial. Better connecting to our inner felt sense can help us to acknowledge our emotional reactions, giving voice to them, thus potentially reducing the effect of chronic stress before it begins to cascade further inwards.

To combat instances of over-thinking outside of the confines of the weekly reflexology sessions, it can be helpful to encourage clients towards introducing more instances of focused relaxation and mindful recognition of their bodily felt sense.

When utilised regularly activities such guided visualisation, regular gentle exercise, and even steeping the feet in a warm water bath, can all promote more relaxed right brained feeling states; helping to quieten the busy mind, and bring the attention back to the here and now. Additionally the increasingly popular concept of mindfulness can prove helpful to many reflexology clients.

Understanding Mindfulness

"Walk as though you are kissing the ground with your feet." - Thích Nhất Hạnh

Mindfulness might be described as paying attention in a particular way, on purpose, and in the present moment. Developing mindfulness practice can sometimes help clients to overcome and combat negative automatic thinking, which can lead to further states of physiological stress and anxiety. The roots of mindfulness are linked most closely to Buddhist philosophy. Today, mindfulness is recommended as a therapeutic intervention by the Department of Health (UK) and by the guidelines set down by NICE (National Institute for Clinical Excellence) as favouring both health and well-being positively. Mindfulness practices can include meditation, awareness of breath and body, listening to music, or even walking. Mindfulness can be a positive tool for stress management because the principles are easily learned, can be used at virtually any time, and can quickly yield positive results.

Benefits of Mindfulness Practice

- Increased instances of calm and relaxation

- Higher levels of energy and enthusiasm for living

- Increased self-confidence and self-acceptance

- Reduced possibility of experiencing stress, depression, anxiety, chronic pain, addiction or low immune efficiency

- Increased self-compassion and compassion for the self, others and the planet

- Focused towards becoming more attentive to the bodily felt sense, mindfulness interventions can help to calm and quiet the busy human mind.

There are many paths encourage mindfulness.

Just Be!

Mindfulness can be incorporated into just about every aspect of our lives, from cleaning our teeth, to walking the dog or taking a stroll. How many people drive along the same road to work each day, but miss the beauty of the changing seasons? How many people eat, but never taste their food? How many hear their friends, family or work colleagues, but never really listen? Mindfulness is concerned with becoming more attentive to the environment in which we reside, and our sensory reactions to it. Mindfulness is in essence about paying more attention!

Meditation

Meditation can bring many benefits and has been one of the most popular and traditional ways to achieve a state of mindfulness for centuries. Meditation often becomes easier with practice, but it need not be difficult for beginners. Simply encourage your client to find a comfortable place free of distractions, and begin to quiet their mind. Focusing initially on a flickering candle flame or a guided meditation can be useful for beginners.

Deep Breathing

"Feelings come and go like clouds in a windy sky. Conscious breathing is my anchor." - Thích Nhất Hạnh

Mindfulness can be as simple as breathing. One of the easiest ways to experience a state of mindfulness is to focus on the breath itself. Breathing from the belly rather than the chest, and trying to breathe in through the nose and out through the mouth. Focusing on the sound and rhythm of the breath, especially when upset, can have a calming effect, and help us to remain grounded in the present moment. It is impossible to think too much when the focus of the mind is on the breath!

Music

Clients might benefit from listening to soothing slow-tempo new-age or classical music. Focusing on the sound and vibration of the notes and perhaps any feelings the music brings to the surface can help keep clients connected in the experience. If other thoughts creep into the head, clients might simply acknowledge them, gently bringing the attention back to the current moment and the music.

Observing Thoughts

Many anxious people find it difficult to stop the rapid stream of thoughts running through their mind, and the idea of trying to sit quietly and meditate — holding off the onslaught of narrative can actually cause more stress. If this sounds like your client, the mindfulness exercise of observing thoughts might be more suited to them.

Rather than working against the narrative running in the head, clients can sit back and simply 'observe' their thoughts. As clients begin to observe, they may find the mind naturally quieting, and the inner narrative becoming less prominent.

Journaling

Some clients might find journaling a helpful way of processing their thoughts. Often just acknowledging the way we feel, by writing it down, can help to reduce the intensity of any associated thought or related anxiety.

Summary

Understanding the manner in which some of our wider therapeutic interactions and recommendations might be impacting our reflexology clients is important not only in order to encourage our own professional development, but also to better ensure we are more able to engage with our clients ethically, empathically and congruently.

The reflexology practitioner who thinks they know best on how to accurately interpret a client is a potentially dangerous and unethical practitioner. It is vitally important to remember, the only true expert in the clients unique life and experiencing, is the client.

The role of the professional reflexologist, particularly when attempting to deal with emotional content, is simply to touch, educate and inform clients using their therapist's bank of knowledge. Practitioners who engage in this manner are far more able to promote increased client self awareness, feelings of autonomy and self-directed change.

The inclusion of reflective responses, particularly when used to help clients become more familiar with their own bodily felt sense, can often prove to be quite transformative. Clients can become aware, sometimes for the first time in many years, exactly *where* their emotional stress is physiologically located, and through the incorporation of mindfulness principles can begin to take steps towards becoming more conscious of, and connected to, their own everyday felt sense responses.

Connected human beings are often happier and healthier human beings.

That is mind, body, spirit.

Relational Reflexology

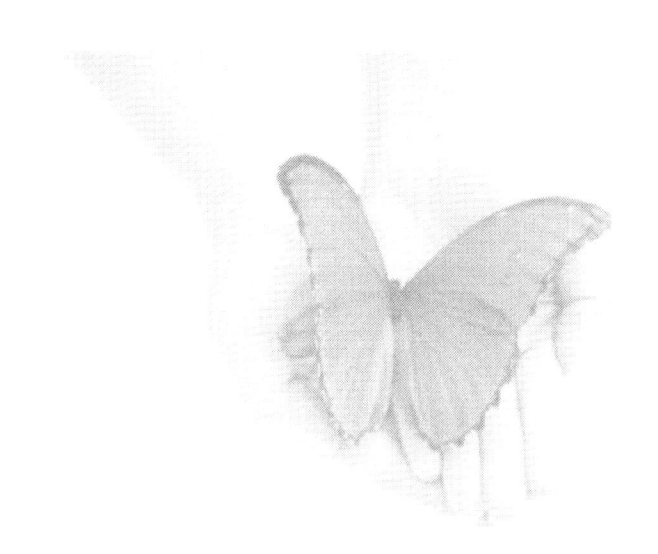

Externalising in Reflexology
Giving Emotions Shapes and Colours

"Emotion always has its roots in the unconscious and manifests itself in the body."

- Irene Claremont de Castillejo

Externalising is a concept first introduced to the field of family therapy in the early 1980s. When an individuals' problem has become *internalized*, a person can come to believe something is really wrong with them, or that *they* are the real source of the problem. Within a reflexology context also some forms of *externalisation* can occur. It is not unusual, for instance, for clients experiencing long term, chronic illness to come to a place where they have accepted they are physiologically *broken*. The practice of owning (internalising) a health condition, accepting it as part of ones being, is certainly not uncommon. For example, many practitioners are likely to have heard comments such as:

"My headaches mean it is difficult for me to ..."
"It's because of my chronic fatigue I can't ..."
"I couldn't find time to meditate/relax this week because..."
"I tried to cut back on the fizzy drinks, but I couldn't help myself ..."

Undoubtedly chronic health conditions are entirely real and wholly experienced. However, if a client comes to truly believe their illness has become a natural part of who they are, then it can also become more challenging to accept the possibility of experiencing a healthier future. The nature of the therapeutic relationship provides reflexology clients not only with a listening ear and emotional support, but it can also be used to provide specific therapeutic interventions and information, capable of promoting the 'externalisation' of clients feelings and frustrations.

Externalising language

The verbal language used by clients to describe their condition can often manifest as containing an *internalised* element. As already mentioned clients can often refer to *my* headaches/migraines/IBS/ME, etc. It can therefore be helpful to encourage *externalisation* during any verbal interactions. In such instances practitioners can simply opt to refer to *the* headaches/migraine, etc. Neutral language such as this (with no ownership) can help to distance the person from the condition, and even help to remind a client of a previous existence without the condition. This stance can in turn help the client to focus on interventions and strategies which might help to impact the now more externalised condition.

Externalisation and Information

As an example, consider the migraine client unaware that four cans of diet coke everyday might be impacting the function of their liver (liver meridian links to blood/flow of Qi (circulation) eyes/headache/migraine). The practitioner who takes time to explain the function of the liver and the associated importance of blood detoxification, for instance, is helping the client to better consider their condition. Information such as this can help to distance the condition from the client, and to present a context for invoking future change.

Externalisation and Guided Visualisation

Helping our clients to develop the skills required to reconnect more fully with their own body **felt sense** can often help to promote change. Clients carrying emotional burdens can often find they think constantly, and repetitively, in turn the brain interprets this constant inner chit chat as fear, and the HPA can be activated almost constantly. Finding ways to calm this innate psychosomatic response can be helpful. Externalising visualisations can be utilised in those instances where when a client has directly acknowledged a feeling of tension or anxiety, perhaps in the chest, abdominal, neck or shoulder area.

Acknowledgments such as these typically occur either directly because of a reflexology body reflection, or because of verbal communications.

Visualisation Exercise

- Ask your client to close their eyes and try to imagine any feelings they are experiencing - be they physical or emotional - as a **colour**. Ask what the colour is?

- Perhaps your client would like to now also like to define a **shape** - is the shape hard or soft - large of small - ask the client for more detail but try not to push too far - use you own intuition to try and read when the detail is stalling, and move on.

- Now ask your client where the shape is **residing** in the body. Client's nearly always to refer to their chest, solar plexus area, or lower abdomen.

- Next ask the client to visualise the shape **emerging** somehow from inside the body to the outside - they may wish to visualise a trap door opening in the area they have identified. Clients can now either visualise the shape floating in the air, or hold it in their hand.

At this point you have helped the client do two things: identify their **felt sense**, and temporarily **externalise** the emotion. There is no requirement to attach a name or narrative to the shape. The shape now simply represents the weight of the emotions carried by the client.

- Now ask the client to take a deep breath and ask how they are feeling? Many clients will report feeling *lighter*, whilst others might say they can *breathe easier*.

- Finally you may wish to ask the client if they would like to **send the shape/feeling away,** temporarily, perhaps attached to a balloon floating off into space.

Summary

The client exposed to directive relaxation and focusing techniques is provided with a therapeutic tool they can also utilise in their everyday environment. Tools such as these encourage more attentiveness towards the physiological felt sense. Any increased contact with the felt sense and gradual realigning of mind and body can help to promote more frequent states of inner calm, and therefore more frequent states of physiological and psychological homeostasis

Externalisation of a condition or feeling, either through language, appropriate information, or guided intervention can help to promote better understanding, a new context, and a path of possible change for reflexology clients.

Developing a Therapeutic Vocabulary in Reflexology

"The limits of my language are the limits of my world."

- Ludwig Wittgenstein

I would define myself principally as a professional reflexologist *(who happens to hold a counselling degree).* By the time I applied to start counsellor training I had already been in reflexology practice nearly three years. I had long since worked out there existed a huge number of struggling individuals, sliding between the medical/psychological support cracks, many of whom seemed to be sliding directly into my reflexology practice. Undoubtedly my initial motivation was to add depth to my holistic work.

Perhaps though, one of the most beneficial elements I gained from completing a counselling degree was the ability to more objectively consider what might be happening within the confines of my reflexology consulting room. I certainly gained a new perspective on how some of our wider therapeutic interactions might be impacting clients. I also developed a renewed and heightened respect for the subtleties, complexities, and possibilities existing within the supportive reflexology package.

Additionally, I became more familiar with the therapeutic language most commonly utilised to define some of those complexities.

CAM – Define Thyself

As a growing CAM industry, reflexology is understandably required to better define, and justify more precisely, any therapeutic worth the modality may offer. Clients receiving complementary therapies can often report multi-dimensional shifts in well-being that seem to go way beyond resolution of the original presenting symptoms.

Within our industry there are some reflexology practitioners who closely identify with a non-directive (ambience centred) form of practice, whilst another group may identify with a more directive (client-centred) form of practice. Many of the more directive practitioners will already be comfortable and familiar with the complex nature of many presenting reflexology clients, and many will be engaging, probably quite naturally, on such a multi-dimensional level.

Certainly, there are many excellent reflexology practitioners already offering effective therapeutic relationships, and providing appropriate information to clients, but how many practitioners are able to more fully define their interventions and interactions with clients?

How Does Developing a Therapeutic Vocabulary Help?

- Developing a therapeutic vocabulary can benefit both the professional practitioner, and indeed the wider reputation of our modality.

- Developing an understanding of therapeutic terms can help practitioners to reflect more objectively on what might be occurring within the confines of their reflexology consulting rooms, and to provide a more open context in which to consider how the reflexology package might be impacting clients.

- Developing an understanding of therapeutic terms can also help to more positively (and accurately) promote the modality. Adopting a therapeutic language, for example, can prove immensely helpful when practitioners come into contact with medical and/or psychological professionals, or may find themselves asked to promote the modality more publicly (radio/magazine articles, etc).

Only a handful of professional reflexologists are ever likely be offered the opportunity to engage in a clinically based type research study, yet, those of us in private practice constitute the much larger majority of professional practitioners. We are then, in essence, the ground troops in reflexology and certainly *we* are responsible for much of the reputation our modality continues to develop. At the top of this article I referred to a large number of struggling individuals often choosing to utilise reflexology in their quest to improve health and wellbeing. Reflexology (in all its various forms) undoubtedly provides therapeutic support to many thousands of clients, and our modality is certainly deserving of wider professional recognition.

One way practitioners can promote our industry, and support the professional associations challenged with steering the modality through some fairly choppy political waters, is to begin to champion the inclusion of a more widely recognised therapeutic vocabulary; one capable of describing the innately multi-dimensional nature of our therapeutic modality.

Common Therapeutic Terms

Autonomy

Philosophy – *the doctrine that the individual human will is, or ought to be governed only by its own principles and laws.*

Autonomy is important within a therapeutic context because the concept is central to promoting self-directed change in clients. In terms of general health care many client have adopted an entirely passive stance – in essence giving away responsibility for their health to outside influences. As clients develop more autonomy, so they also tend to develop a renewed sense of control in their life and experiencing.

Beneficence

The principle of beneficence means acting in the best interests of the client, based on professional assessment. Beneficence is an ethical principle concerned with directing our attention towards working within our limits of professional competence. Ensuring that client's best interests are maintained requires systematic monitoring of practice and outcomes, by the best available means.

An obligation to act in the best interests of a client may become of paramount importance when engaging with clients whose capacity for autonomy is diminished, because of immaturity, lack of understanding, extreme distress, or other significant personal constraints.

Congruence

Within a therapeutic context congruence can be defined as one of ways of being associated with the core conditions required to form effective therapeutic relationships, proposed by the humanistic psychologist and founder of person-centred theory, Carl Rogers (1951).

Congruence refers to state of being in which the practitioner attempts to present as entirely real or genuine, within the therapeutic relationship.

Disclosure

The act or process of revealing or uncovering.

Within a therapeutic context disclosure refers to the personal and emotional material clients choose to bring to the consulting room, and share with the practitioner. When clients disclose information they are in essence inviting the practitioner into their unique personal emotional realm.

Empathy

Identification with, and understanding of, another's situation, feelings, and/or motives. Empathic understanding can demonstrate the practitioner's ability to appreciate the client's unique frame of reference.

Existential

1. Of, relating to, or dealing with existence.

2. Based on unique experience.

Existentialism is a philosophical outlook that stresses the importance of free will, freedom of choice, and personal responsibility.

Externalising

1. To attribute to outside causes.

2. To project or attribute (inner conflicts or feelings) to external circumstances or causes.

Within a therapeutic context externalising can help clients to re-define their present stance, and provide a more appropriate context for promoting autonomy and self-directed change. Often the information and support provided by practitioners can help clients to externalise their problems or condition. Providing appropriate information can help to separate the problem/condition from the person.

Homeostasis

1. The tendency of a system, especially the physiological system of higher animals, to maintain internal stability, owing to the co-ordinated response of its parts to any situation or stimulus tending to disturb its normal condition or function.

2. A state of psychological equilibrium obtained when tension or a drive has been reduced or eliminated.

HPA Axis

The hypothalamic-pituitary-adrenal axis is a complex set of interactions between the hypothalamus (emotion/brain), the pituitary gland (brain) and the adrenal glands (body). The HPA axis helps to regulate temperature, digestion, immune system, mood, sexuality and metabolism. It is also a major part of the system that controls our reactions to stress, trauma and injury, the fight or flight response.

Internal Supervisor

Carl Rogers wrote of a dawning realisation – that moment when the individual believes that they have within them the capability of deciding their own values and judgements. Practitioners who learn to trust their own inner supervisor (principally resulting from practitioner self development, integrating high levels of appropriate information and remaining respectful of ethical principles) tend to develop less reliance on the evaluation and opinions of others, and more faith and belief in their own judgement.

Multi-Dimensional

Of, relating to, or having several dimensions.

Within a supportive reflexology context multi-dimensional is used to contextualise both the unique phenomenological experience of individual client, and also the various elements identified within the reflexology package as containing the potential to influence clients, and therefore promote change.

Non-Maleficence

Non-maleficence is an ethical principle related to avoiding sexual, financial, emotional, sexual or any other form of client exploitation; avoiding incompetence or malpractice; not providing services when unfit to do so, due to illness, personal circumstances or intoxication. The practitioner holds an ethical responsibility to strive to mitigate any potential harm to clients.

Person-Centred Theory

Person-Centred Therapy (PCT) was developed by the humanistic psychologist Carl Rogers in the 1940s. The theoretical core of PCT leans towards practitioners developing a more personal relationship with their client. Person-Centred theory promotes the concept that clients remain the only experts in their life and experiencing.

Phenomenology

A philosophy, or method of research inquiry based on the premise that reality consists of objects and events as they are perceived or understood in human consciousness, and not of anything independent of human consciousness. The perceptions and reactions of the individual are always entirely unique.

Psychoneuroimmunology

The scientific study of interactions between psychological factors (mind), the central nervous system (brain) and the immune system (body), as modulated by the neuroendocrine system.

The study focuses on emotional, and other psychological states, capable of impacting immune and endocrine responses and rendering the individual less or more susceptible to disease, and vice versa.

Psychosomatic

1. Of a physical illness or other condition caused or aggravated by a mental factor such as internal conflict or stress.

2. Relating to the interaction of mind (psycho) and body (soma).

Relational

1. Of, or arising from kinship.

2. Indicating or constituting relation.

Within a therapeutic context relational can be defined as an interaction between two individuals; specifically the interaction between the practitioner and client.

Relational Depth

"A state of profound contact and engagement between two people, in which each person is fully real with the Other, and able to understand and value the Other's experiences at a high level." Rogers (1951)

Supervision

Many professionals engage in supportive supervision. Unfortunately the concept is presently undervalued by the general complementary therapy world. Supportive supervision can help to build confidence in practitioners, and help to promote development of the practitioners own internal supervisor.

Perhaps, rather than looking to our insurance policies for guidance on when and when not to treat, practitioners might fare better by looking towards professional supervision to gain more clarity and direction.

Until such a time as our profession can offer supervision from within the industry, practitioners may benefit from engaging with a supportive local counsellor/supervisor.

Therapeutic Relationship

A working or helping professional alliance.

Unconditional Positive Regard

A phrase coined by Carl Rogers (1951). UPR can be defined as absolute acceptance and support of the individual, regardless of what the individual says or does. UPR is really about finding value in all fellow human beings.

Summary

Reflexologists are certainly not counsellors, but we do have much in common with our talking therapy colleagues. Whilst undoubtedly reflexology practitioners have no requirement to understand for example, theoretical information regarding the development of the self, or personality, we certainly can make good use of existing information relating to therapeutic relationships, ethics and boundaries, and indeed some of the terms more commonly used to define and describe individual client phenomenology.

Initially, some of the terms may seem overly complex and confusing. Try to remember, it is likely you once felt the same way about a reflexology foot map!

Relational Reflexology

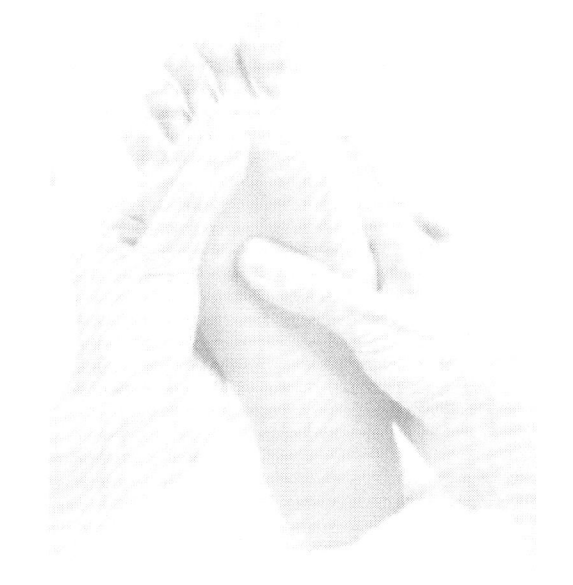

Reflexology and the Whole Person
Interstitial Cystitis

"The part can never be well, unless the whole is well"

- Plato

Interstitial Cystitis (IC) is a chronic inflammation of the bladder wall, sometimes also diagnosed as Painful Bladder Syndrome (PBS). Symptoms can include mild to severe pressure and discomfort, urinary frequency and/or the frequent urge to urinate. Interstitial cystitis is not a bacterial infection, although the symptoms can feel similar. It is believed the ratio of women to men in the U.K. developing the conditions stands at around 9:1, however, it has been suggested a large percentage of men may be alternatively misdiagnosed with conditions such as prostatitis.

Interstitial cystitis is a deeply distressing, debilitating and painful disorder. Epidemiological studies have indicated it can take on average five to seven years to obtain an accurate diagnosis of of IC, and that many clients score badly on quality of life studies. IC clients can experience severe pelvic pain and the need to urinate as often as every 10 to 15 minutes, day and night, meaning many can become housebound and/or unable to work or care for their families.

The Normally Functioning Bladder

Under normal conditions urine flows from the kidney to the bladder via the ureters. The bladder is mostly constructed of muscle, to allow for expansion as urine collects. The urethra is responsible for allowing urine to pass from the bladder. The sphincter of the urethra normally remains closed to prevent urine from leaking. During urination the sphincter relaxes and opens, allowing urine to pass from the body. Both the bladder and urethra have a specialised lining called the epithelium.

The epithelium essentially forms a barrier between the urine and the bladder muscle, helping to prevent bacteria from sticking to the bladder wall.

What Causes Interstitial Cystitis?

The cause of interstitial cystitis is presently unknown. There are currently no absolute defining tests to confirm the presence of the condition therefore diagnosis is generally made by a process of elimination. Indications stemming from research, however, suggest the condition may be linked to:

- A defect in the bladder epithelium
- A specific type of inflammatory cell (mast cell) releasing histamine and other chemicals
- The presence of something in the urine capable of damaging the bladder
- Changes to the nerves responsible for carrying bladder sensations
- An autoimmune disorder

Psychoneuroimmunology

Psychoneuroimmunology (PNI) is a relatively young branch of scientific study attempting to examine the subtle interactions between human psychological processes, and the function of the nervous, immune and endocrine systems. The main emphasis in PNI is to portray that complex biological systems are in essence integrated therefore the field focuses on studying the relationship between systems, rather than the study of individual components.

PNI considers connections between how stress and the mind can influence the physical body, and vice versa. PNI also supports a holistic rationale stating mind and body are undoubtedly intertwined and connected, and, that the experiences and perceptions of the individual can directly affect the body's wider function.

The principles of psychoneuroimmunology are closely linked to the study of *epigenetics*:

"Epigenetic's literally means "above" or "on top of" genetics. It refers to external modifications to DNA that turn genes "on" or "off." These modifications do not change the DNA sequence, but instead, they affect how cells "read" genes." (livescience.com)

Interstitial Cystitis and Chronic Stress and Anxiety

"When it comes to a stressful emergency, a bladder means a lot of sloshy dead weight to carry in your sprint across the savanna. The answer is obvious: empty that bladder!" (Sapolsky, 2004)

Research has demonstrated that chronic stress can alter gene activity in immune cells before they reach the bloodstream. Prolonged activation of the fight or flight response can result in the production of white blood cells (produced in the bone marrow) more inflammatory than would normally be expected upon release. These cells are, in essence, primed and ready to defend the body against a perceived external threat.

Stress within this context can be defined as:

"Stress that triggers the sympathetic nervous system, commonly known as the fight-or-flight response, and stimulates the production of new blood cells. While this response is important for survival, prolonged activation over an extended period of time can have negative effects on health." (neurosciencenews.com)

Considering interstitial cystitis specifically, research has demonstrated:

"There is an important correlation between interstitial cystitis and rheumatic, auto-immune and chronic inflammatory diseases." (Lorenzo and Gomez, 2004)

and:

"No data support a direct causal role of autoimmune reactivity in the pathogenesis of interstitial cystitis. Indirect evidence, however, does support a possible autoimmune nature of interstitial cystitis, such as the strong female preponderance and the clinical association between interstitial cystitis and other known autoimmune diseases within patients and their families." (Van de Merwe, 2007)

Interstitial Cystitis and Traditional Chinese Medicine

Within the context of TCM Interstitial cystitis has no absolute defined classical definition, but may be more loosely classified as a deficiency condition, principally linked to kidney or spleen energy.

The **kidney**, **bladder**, **spleen** and **stomach** meridians each run into the **feet**.

Stimulation of the feet according to TCM promotes the movement of blood and Qi around the body. The Ancient Chinese described the feet as the roots of the body.

According to TCM the **kidney** and **bladder** meridians are associated with:

- The Jing - inherited genetically at conception. Jing resides in the kidney and from there flows throughout the body via the meridian system
- Jing provides the vital organs with the energy to function properly and efficiently
- The urinary system
- The emotions of sustained fear and fright
- Physical and emotional exhaustion

The **spleen** and **stomach** meridians are considered to be associated with:

- Spleen energy is responsible for extracting nutrients from the food we consume and converting that energy into blood and Qi.

- According to TCM, pensiveness is considered to result from thinking too much, or excessive mental stimulation and the organ most at risk is the spleen.

- A deficiency of spleen Qi can result in feelings of worry, fatigue, lethargy, and an inability to concentrate.

The Client

Marc came to see me some four years after first displaying symptoms of Interstitial cystitis – his call prompted by a verbal recommendation from a local G.P. Marc's symptoms initially displayed whilst he was attending university, and he was further able to identify it was during his daily commute that problems first became noticeable. Since the onset of his symptoms Marc had been under the care of three different urologists, before finally opting to pay privately for a third and final consultation, and associated testing.

Marc's Words:

"I'd visited three urologists across a four year period, and been through numerous painful procedures, including a biopsy and a bladder stretch. I was given several different medications, including powerful anti-biotics, oyxbutynin, transdermal patches, tolteradine, trospium and solifenacin. I also did lots of bladder training, which I was assured would solve the problem, and when no improvement came, it was suggested I simply wasn't doing the exercises. Additionally I cut out caffeine and fruit juices from my diet, and reduced other sources of dietary caffeine, such as chocolate."

The Initial Consultation

Marc is a quiet, softly spoken, intelligent and highly capable individual. Marc revealed during our initial consultation how deeply distressing and limiting his condition had become, and how it was now affecting every aspect of his life. His urge to urinate was almost constant, and the discomfort he experienced excruciating. None of the medication seemed to help and Marc was utterly exhausted. After being discharged from urology for the final time, Marc was offered a referral to psychiatry – a referral he considered to be deeply offensive.

Marc initially enquired about the possibility of hypnotherapy to help with his condition, but after our first consultation appointment, I suggested reflexology might be a more beneficial option.

During our initial consultation I was to explain to Marc the principles of TCM and how his condition might be classified (kidney-bladder-fear/spleen-stomach-pensivness). This information offered to Marc the concept that his ever present daily distress may be exacerbating the condition.

I was additionally able to explain the principles of psychoneuroimmunology, and the associated function of the HPA axis. This information additionally highlighted the scientific concept suggesting his mind and thought processes were certainly capable of impacting him physiologically.

This form of verbal explanation is absolutely crucial when attempting any form of psychosomatic work with clients. Marc revealed he felt deeply offended when his consultant suggested he should visit the psychiatrist – considering the suggestion to suppose he must have mental health issues. Certainly, in Marc's case, this was absolutely not the case. Clients rarely imagine their physical symptoms. The unfortunate separation between mind and body existing within western medicine means clients are often not given an appropriate context from which to better understand their condition. It is imperative reflexology clients such as Marc, are provided with such a context; as such an offering can provide a potential new path to follow towards better health.

Marc certainly did not require psychiatric medication rather he needed to become more familiar and attentive to his own internal thought patterns, stress responses and general levels of anxiety. There is a misconception existing, suggesting individuals who experience high levels of stress or anxiety must therefore have mental health problems – this is simply *not* the case. Many of our reflexology clients are simply worriers, troubled by a high level of internal chit chat and narrative. Marc's determination to overcome his condition meant he was still working full-time, despite his symptoms, and if you had met him back then it is highly unlikely you would consider him to be a man experiencing anxiety. He certainly hid his feelings well.

Within a reflexology context practitioners who choose to engage in this type of work can potentially utilise and promote the inclusion of mindfully based interventions, or suggest guided mediation, within any treatment plan. In some instances (when the anxiety seems to be more deep seated) it may be beneficial to refer the client for counselling support, to run alongside reflexology.

The Sessions

- Marc received reflexology on a weekly basis, across several months. The most noticeable factor Marc displayed physiologically during the sessions was pronounced shaking and muscle tremors. These tremors (possibly either linked to excessive levels of adrenaline in the blood - or deep-seated emotional content with the tissues) began to subside as the weeks progressed.

- Marc received a full and firm reflexology treatment at each session, with extra attention given to the brain, adrenal and urinary reflexes.

- Marc was additionally able to use the space and confines of the therapeutic relationship to talk about his experience; his pain, his frustration, his fears regarding the condition, and his levels of physical and emotional exhaustion.

- Marc agreed to steep his feet in hot water daily to further promote good circulation, and to encourage more instances of daily relaxation.

- Marc also began to take note of his own internal stress responses, endeavouring to become more consciously aware of his inner reactions and feelings.

Some three months into reflexology treatment Marc's urgency to urinate had begun to subside significantly. The real turning point came when Marc was asked to go and price a job for his employer. Now better able to undertake longer car journeys, Marc agreed to the challenge and set off, comfortable in the knowledge he could manage the journey, and knowing there was a public toilet in the car park he planned to use on arrival.

When Marc arrived at the car park, he soon became aware the public toilet was closed for refurbishment. Marc later reported his own observation of the event – stating that he felt immediate panic on viewing the closed sign, and quickly thereafter became aware of the familiar necessity to urinate.

In that moment, Marc became fully and consciously aware that his feelings of fear and panic preceded his requirement to urinate. Marc still attends for reflexology on a monthly basis, and the condition is now under control. He rarely experiences symptoms, and feels much more able to control his reactions to his environment.

Summary

The reflexology package can be transformative for many clients. During a session clients benefit from:

- Physical stimulation of over 7000 nerve ending in the feet, each one communicating directly with the brain.

- Stimulation of the circulation.

- The therapeutic benefit of touch, widely researched and proven to be beneficial, both psychologically and physiologically.

- Emotional support stemming from the therapeutic relationship.

- Increased levels of autonomy and self directed change stemming from appropriate information.

Marc initially attended for reflexology as an emotionally distressed and deeply frustrated individual. The nature of the therapeutic relationship provided a safe space in which Marc was able to disclose his feelings, and to discuss his frustration. Additionally, Marc was able to receive – and therefore respond to – clinical and philosophical information I was able to provide; information which ultimately promoted the concepts of client autonomy, and self-directed change.

The beautician, or spa type reflexologist, may well be entirely capable of inducing an hour of deep relaxation in their clients, but I am *not* a beautician. I am a professional reflexologist and therapist, and the clients who visit me often do so because of chronic illness.

It is worth remembering the only person who can really reduce frequent, prolonged activation of the hypothalamus-pituitary-adrenal axis – is the client.

My role as a professional reflexologist is to touch, support and educate my clients, so that they are better informed, and therefore more capable of invoking long term change.

That is mind, body, spirit.

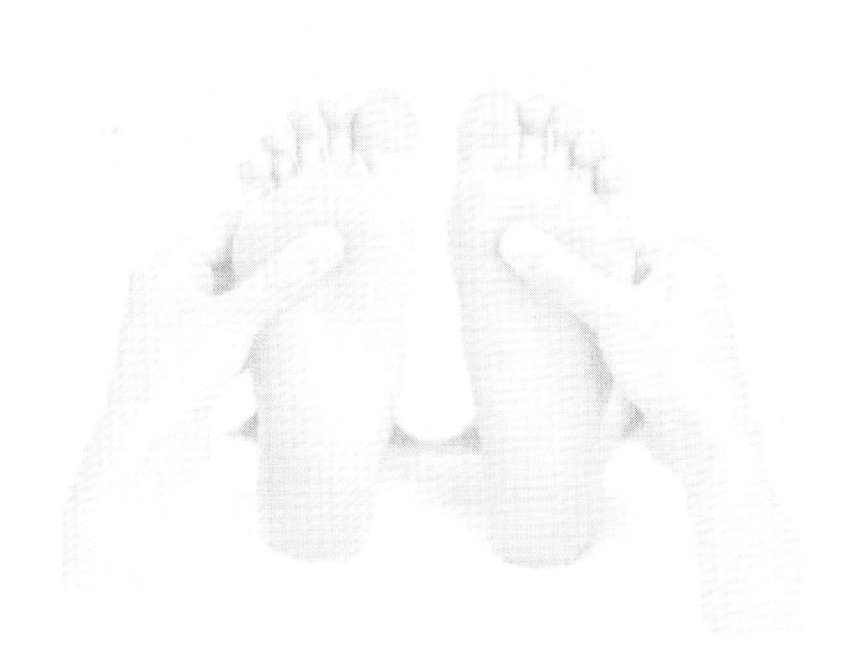

Relational Reflexology

Reflexology and the Whole Person
Chronic Headache and Migraine

"Therefore it appears to me necessary to every physician to be skilled in the ways of nature,
and strive to know, if he would wish to perform his duties,
what man is in relation to the articles of food and drink, and to his other occupations,
and what are the effects of each of them to every one."

- Hippocrates

Chronic headache and migraine are distressing and often debilitating conditions. To achieve a medical diagnosis of chronic headache or migraine clients need to report pain across 15 days a month. Most clients are prescribed a cocktail of topical analgesia and prophylactic (preventative) medication. Chronic migraine can present as a stand-alone condition, or can display in conjunction with either cluster headaches and/or ice pick headaches. Additionally clients can often describe feeling a foggy, or fuzzy painful head. Some clients experience less common types of headache, similar to the one presented later in this article.

Over Use of Analgesia

Medication-induced headaches are caused by overuse of painkillers or triptan medication (triptans are a class of drugs used to treat migraine or cluster headaches). These types of headaches can be defined as headaches occurring daily, or on most days. Medication-induced headache is the third most common cause of headache after migraine and tension-type headache.

The Migraine Trust states:

"The extent to which frequent usage of analgesics or triptans causes problems seems to vary from one drug to another, and in all likelihood varies considerably from one patient to another. Our experience is that over-usage of ergotamine, triptans and opiate based medications (from codeine-based products up to morphine) tend to cause problems most frequently, with paracetamol and non-steroidal anti-inflammatory drugs (NSAIDs) such as aspirin, ibuprofen or naproxen less likely to do so. The International Headache Society criteria for medication overuse reflects this, with opiate or triptan over-usage defined as ten days or more per month, whereas over-usage of paracetamol or NSAID is deemed to be present when these drugs are used 15 or more days per month."

Pressure placed upon the liver due to excessive prolonged medication consumption can impact blood quality. In essence the liver might be likened to large chemical processing factory. When the liver becomes *'overworked'*, due to repeatedly encountering the chemical components of many medications, wider knock on effects seem to present in associated parts and organs of the body.

The Greater Occipital Nerve

Most of the feeling in the back and top of the head is transmitted to the brain by the two greater occipital nerves. The nerves emerge from the cervical vertebrae in the upper neck. The two occipital nerves extend up and across the back of the head and into the scalp, sometimes reaching as far forward as the forehead. Irritation of one or both of the nerves can cause a shooting, electric, or tingling pain located on one side of the scalp. Sometimes the pain can radiate toward the eye. Problems can sometimes occur spontaneously, or as the result of a pinched nerve root, caused by tight neck muscles or arthritis, for example.

Additionally, injury or surgery to the scalp or skull can result in irritation of the occipital nerve(s). Many types of headache, including migraine, predominately involve the back of one side of the head. Patients with headaches of this type are often diagnosed with chronic headache or migraines involving the greater occipital nerve, rather than occipital neuralgia, which is much less common.

Chronic Headache/Migraine and Traditional Chinese Medicine

"Chronic headaches more often accompany internal disharmonies. Severe headaches are usually signs of excess, while slight, annoying headaches are usually signs of deficiency. The organ most associated with headaches is the liver, because liver qi often rises when the liver is in disharmony." (Kaptchuk, 2000)

Chronic headache and migraine within a TCM context tend to be viewed as excessive conditions. However, there are three more specific differentiations of headaches according to TCM:

- Headache due to invasion of pathogenic wind in the meridians.
- Headache due to upsurge of liver yang.
- Headache due to deficiency of Qi and blood.

The liver meridian runs into the feet and big toes. Stimulation of the feet according to TCM promotes the movement of blood and Qi around the body. The Ancient Chinese described the feet as the roots of the body. According to TCM the liver meridian is associated with:

- The blood
- The free flow of Qi around the body
- The muscles
- The eyes
- The emotions: anger and irritation

The Psychology

Whilst reflexologists are not counsellors, practitioners do often find themselves listening to their clients. Dealing with chronic pain can be utterly exhausting, both physiologically and psychologically. As a result conditions such as chronic headache and migraine can impact across many areas of the individual's life. The International Institute for the Study of Pain (Traue, et al), define pain as:

"An unpleasant sensory and emotional experience, associated with actual or potential tissue damage, or described in terms of such damage."

Going on to state:

"Pain is often accompanied by strong emotions. It is perceived not only as a sensation described with words such as burning, pressing stabbing or cutting, but also as an emotional experience (feeling) with words such as agonising, cruel, terrible and excruciating."

Owning Illness

I have personally yet to meet a long term chronic headache or migraine client at consultation who has not already come to believe they are physiologically *broken*. Perhaps this stance is adopted when an individual reaches the point of believing *'if the highest qualified expert in the land (the neurologist) isn't able to fix it … then surely nothing can?'* Perhaps this is the point at which one gives up hope?

The practice of owning a health condition and accepting it as part of ones being is not uncommon. For example, many practitioners will have heard phrases such as; "My headaches mean it's difficult for me to …" or, "It's because of my chronic fatigue I can't"…? Undoubtedly these deeply distressing and painful conditions are entirely real and wholly experienced. However, when a client comes to truly believe their illness has become a natural part of who they are, then it can also become more challenging to visualise a real existence without the presence of the condition. The nature of the therapeutic relationship can provide an appropriate context in which practitioners are able to offer a listening ear and emotional support. The therapeutic relationship can also be used to provide appropriate information able to promote existential change in clients.

Sarah – The Client

Sarah came to see me some two years after a clinical diagnosis of chronic cluster headaches affecting only the left eye. Typically, Sarah could be woken up to ten times a night by an excruciating, burning pain in her eyeball. Sarah was under the care of a consultant neurologist, and had been prescribed both daily prophylactic and topical analgesic medication. Some nights were better than others, but Sarah reported in over two years she had only experienced a handful of nights without an attack. During our initial consultation the impact of Sarah's condition became clear. Her left pupil was noticeably dilated, and her eye was generally bloodshot. Sarah looked generally tired, rundown and underweight, but reported to be a happy and fairly contented lady; aside from the headaches she felt all was well in her world and considered her job in social work to be *'sometimes stressful, but very rewarding.'* During the consultation Sarah mentioned she had been following a vegan diet for several years. Sarah additionally reported some mild neck pain and general stiffness.

The Consultation Session

Sarah is a thoughtful, timid, slightly nervous lady in her mid thirties. Her hands have the tendency to fidget; she smiles a lot, and offers compliments freely. Liver energy rising according to TCM is associated with repressed anger and states of agitation and irritation; these were not emotions I was readily picking up from Sarah's language, descriptions or body language. Instead I felt more drawn to focusing on Sarah's diet, and an associated potential deficiency in the blood and Qi because of her vegan diet. Protein influences blood quality (protein is required by the body for cell renewal). Sarah and I discussed her vegan diet, specifically focusing on her protein intake. We also explored a potential link connected to a sleep related drop in blood pressure, and Sarah's general energy levels.

Sarah agreed to do some of her own research and report back her findings. (It can often be helpful to encourage clients to take more responsibility for their body and wider health care. Client research can promote autonomy and self directed change).

The Sessions

At the next session Sarah was able to report she estimated her protein intake was less than 40% of the recommended daily requirement, and she was able to explain how she planned to rectify the situation. I worked on Sarah using reflexology for six weeks initially, performing a full and firm treatment. I gave extra attention to the head/brain, neck, cervical vertebrae, shoulder, liver and adrenals. Additionally, Sarah was asked to steep her feet in hot water daily, a practice often performed prior to reflexology in the East in order to promote stimulation of the blood and to open the pores. Sarah also agreed to use a heated beanbag on her neck daily. Sarah was additionally able to use the space and confines of the therapeutic relationship to talk about her experience; her pain, her fears regarding her condition, and her levels of exhaustion.

Across this six week period Sarah began to report a lessening in the frequency, duration and intensity of the attacks, resulting in a reduction in her use of topical analgesia. During week seven, for the first time, Sarah's pain spontaneously moved from the left to right eye, where it lingered for an additional three weeks. By week twelve Sarah reported one attack across the entire week.

Sarah is now free from prescribed medication, and has been discharged by neurology. The attacks are now consistently limited to one or two occurrences, at or around the time of menstruation. Sarah continues to attend every six weeks for reflexology and upholds her dietary requirements, endeavouring to consume a more balanced diet.

Summary

The information presented towards the top of this blog is a summarised representation of my present personal knowledge regarding chronic headache and migraine. It is from this bank of knowledge I am able drawn upon and educate each individual client. Through presenting relevant information, and allowing the client to choose a meaning which seems appropriate for them, we are able to promote client autonomy. Education and reflective information gathering and exchanges promote self-directed client change. From a psychological perspective this can be viewed as a highly beneficial stance; related to clients potentially regaining some element of control.

Sarah was able to benefit not only from the physical application of reflexology and the support of an empathic practitioner, but also from appropriate education regarding her body and its functions. Sarah was able then to choose a meaning which resonated with her own experience, and act upon the information she gathered. A different client may find a different meaning, and perhaps recognise that neck tension presents the biggest challenge. This client may require referral to an osteopath, chiropractor or masseur for more direct manipulation, to run alongside reflexology. Another client may identify that alcohol or perhaps a toxic diet, compounded by medication are potential contributing factors, and again can benefit from the choice to make changes.

Within my private practice my ethical responsibility requires I work with my clients best interests in mind. As a professional reflexologist I choose to my work entirely holistically. I provide the setting, intervention and appropriate relevant information for each individual client. I engage therapeutically with the whole person.

That is mind, body, spirit.

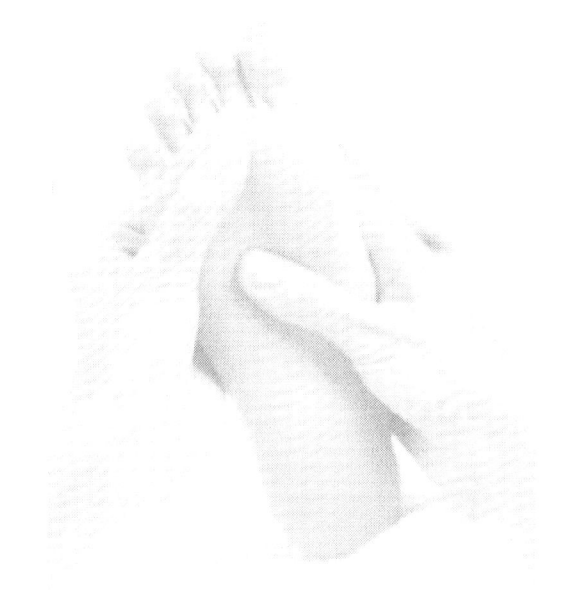

Relational Reflexology

Reflexology and the Whole Person
Vertigo, Tinnitus, and Labyrinthitis

"There is more wisdom in your body than in your deepest philosophy."

- Friedrich Nietzsche

Whilst vertigo, tinnitus, and labyrinthitis are classified separately in a medical definition sense, they do certainly share some overlapping elements in regards to how clients are more widely affected.

More specifically, each of these conditions is closely associated with states of internal anxiety and physical and emotional exhaustion.

Additionally, it is not uncommon for individuals diagnosed with tinnitus to also experience some of the symptoms of vertigo, and vice versa.

The symptoms associated with labyrinthitis might be described more generally as a combination of vertigo and tinnitus.

Clients presenting for reflexology with these types of ear/balance related conditions can be categorised loosely in the following manner:

- Most common in 45-70 age groups.

- Affecting both men and women, but very common in menopausal and post menopausal women.

- Almost always accompanied by feelings of emotional distress and anxiety.

The Inner Ear

The inner ear is mainly responsible for sound detection and balance. The inner ear consists of consists of the **labyrinth**; a hollow cavity in the temporal bone of the skull containing two main parts:

- **The cochlea:** responsible for relaying sound to the brain and hearing - converts sound pressure patterns from the outer ear into electrochemical impulses which are passed on to the brain via the auditory nerve

- **The vestibular system:** fluid-filled channels related to the sense of balance

The Proprioceptive System

The proprioceptive system refers the system responsible for the sense of the position of the various parts of the body, and stands distinct from both exteroception (sense observation relating to the outside world), and interoception (internal body state sense). When an individual is blindfolded for example, he or she knows through *proprioception* if their arm is above their head or hanging by the side of the body.

The sense of proprioception can be disturbed in many disorders, including vertigo. *Sensory* information from the neck is combined with *vestibular* and *visual* information to determine the position of the head on the neck and space around. Abnormal input from proprioceptors in the neck can therefore cause *vertigo*. Like other sensory systems the proprioceptive system involves a pathway from the peripheral nervous system to the thalamus and on to dedicated parts of the cortex.

Vertigo

Vertigo is described as the sensation that the individual, or the environment around them, is moving or spinning. In TCM there certainly exists as link between reproductive hormones and the ears. Additionally, the number of menopausal women entering my therapy room would seem to verify this connection. However, researchers tell us:

"Despite evidence to support the link, the role of the endocrine system in vestibular function and disease is as yet virtually unexplored." (Seemungal, 2001)

There are conditions capable of causing vertigo such as, Ménière's disease, Migraine and Vestibular Neuronitis (an inflammation of the vestibular nerve connecting the ear and brain). Most commonly individuals affected by vertigo report:

- Intense spells of dizziness and loss of balance
- Feelings of nausea
- Emotional distress

Benign Paroxysmsl Positional Vertigo (BPPV)

BPPV is defined as repeated bouts of vertigo brought on as a result of certain head movements. This form of vertigo sometimes responds well to a technique called '*Epley's Manoeuvre*'. It is recommended clients falling into this category are referred back to their GP (who may perform the manoeuvre), or provide a referral to a local physiotherapist or osteopath.

Tinnitus

Tinnitus is defined as any sound the individual is able to hear not stemming from the outside environment. There is currently no definitive medical treatment for the condition. Tinnitus is most commonly described as 'ringing in the ears' although those affected can also report:

- Buzzing, humming, whooshing, hissing, whistling, or a noise moving in time with the pulse (pulsatile tinnitus).
- Emotional distress.

"Tinnitus frequently represents a symptom of an associated disease process. Recent research has employed state-of-the-art imaging and measurement technology to examine tinnitus-related activity in the ear, auditory nerve, and auditory tracts of the brain. These studies have increasingly focused on exploring putative brain-related mechanisms. The complexity of the changes in the nervous system associated with tinnitus might explain why this condition has proved so resistant to treatment." (Han et al., 2009)

It was previously theorised that tinnitus was generated by direct damage to the cochlea (the hearing organ of the inner ear). This stance led to attempts to cure tinnitus by severing the auditory nerve connecting the cochlea to the brain however, this procedure was found to be ineffective, often resulting in a worsening of the individual's symptoms. These findings lead to scientists beginning to consider whether tinnitus was actually being generated by the brain itself.

"Tinnitus generators are theoretically located in the auditory pathway, and such generators and various mechanisms occurring in the peripheral auditory system have been explained in terms of spontaneous otoacoustic emissions, edge theory, and discordant theory. Those present in the central auditory system have been explained in terms of the dorsal cochlear nucleus, the auditory plasticity theory, the crosstalk theory, the somatosensory system, and the limbic and autonomic nervous systems." (Han et al., 2009).

Researchers now suggest tinnitus may manifest as a result of parts of the brain linked to sensory perception becoming *over active*. In its natural state the intricate auditory system should activate in response to sensory input received from the external environment. Because damage to the cochlear (caused by wear and tear, infection or inflammation) can result in a reduction of input to the brain's hearing system, the brain responds by over-compensating for this loss of hearing by spontaneously activating the auditory system *loop*, thus the individual begins to perceive sound where in reality there is none. In essence the brain turns the speaker up!

"The condition arises when hairs in the inner ear are damaged and the brain's auditory neurons fire more frequently, trying to amplify sounds." (Rauschecker et al., 2010)

Labyrinthitis

Labyrinthitis is defined as an inflammation of the inner ear (the labyrinth), affecting the individual's sense of balance and hearing. Experts believe inflammation in this area is most commonly caused by a viral infection, and less commonly a bacterial infection. There is currently no single defining medical treatment for labyrinthitis. Individuals affected by the disorder can report:

- Intense spells of dizziness and loss of balance
- Feeling of nausea
- Hearing loss
- Noise in the ear
- Emotional distress

Autoimmune Inner Ear Disease

Autoimmune sensorineural hearing loss was first highlighted in a research paper (McCabe, 1979) describing oatients whose:

"clinical pattern did not fit with known entities and thus seemed to merit distinctive categorisation."

AIED consists of a syndrome of progressive hearing loss and/or dizziness which is caused by antibodies or immune cells which are attacking the inner ear. It is believed AIED can occur in isolation (labyrinthitis) or as part of other systemic autoimmune disorders. It is estimated up to twenty percent of patients have other autoimmune diseases, such as rheumatoid arthritis or lupus.

"Autoimmune inner ear disease (AIED) is a syndrome of progressive hearing loss and/or dizziness that is caused by antibodies or immune cells which are attacking the inner ear.

In most cases, there is reduction of hearing accompanied by tinnitus (ringing, hissing, roaring) which occurs over a few months. Variants are bilateral attacks of hearing loss and tinnitus that resemble Meniere's disease, and attacks of dizziness accompanied by abnormal blood tests for antibodies. About 50% of patients with AIED have symptoms related to balance (dizziness or unsteadiness). (american-hearing.org).

Other Information

Evidence suggests vitamins A and D, and the minerals iron, and zinc can be low in individuals with hearing disorders. There is also some indication that bioflavonoids and omega-3 fatty acids can yield improvement in individuals with hearing disorders and Meniere's diseases.

Tinnitus, Vertigo, Labyrinthitis and TCM

According to TCM the **kidney** meridian is partnered with the bladder meridian, and the associated sensory organ is the **ears**. Kidney energy is further associated with:

- **Jing** - The Jing is inherited genetically at conception. Jing resides in the kidney and from there flows throughout the body via the meridian system. Jing provides the **vital organs** with the energy to function properly and efficiently.

- The emotions of sustained **fear** and **fright**.

- Physical and emotional **exhaustion**.

In the Neijing Suwen, written around 100 B.C., several potential causes of tinnitus are mentioned.

"Kidney Qi communicates with the ears; when the kidneys are functioning well, the five types of sound can be heard."

The term kidney, as used by the ancient Chinese, refers to a functional system that is difficult to link to specific organs, but is said to involve not only the kidneys, but also the wider endocrine system. Kidney Qi (*linked to longevity*) is believed to weaken with age, and hearing problems, as well as difficulties with other senses, can arise as a result.

The Client Group

The greater majority of individuals who enquire about reflexology in this client group will have already been diagnosed by a GP, or consulted with an ENT (ear, nose and throat) specialist. Western medicine unfortunately had very little to offer this particular group of clients, and so by the time many of these individuals make contact, they will have been dealing with their deeply distressing symptoms for many weeks, and sometimes months.

It is perhaps difficult to imagine how stressful it must be to constantly hear a ringing or buzzing noise, or to feel suddenly unsure about driving after twenty five years behind the wheel. These distressing conditions are entirely capable of stripping an individual of their sense of confidence and existential freedoms. The conditions can rapidly become crippling, and impact *every* area of the individual's life.

Vertigo and labyrinthitis clients will often report they feel they must be alert and vigilant of their every movement - mindful of how they rise from a chair, or lie down in bed. Any sudden jolt, *they fear*, might send them off into a severe spinning episode. Simple tasks, such as shopping, can become difficult because bright tungsten lights inside many supermarkets can set off the dizzy feelings. The tinnitus client meanwhile finds it difficult to sleep, or to concentrate on anything much outside of the noises constantly in their ears. The poor labyrinthitis client is unfortunately served a double dose - dizzy and ringing. The conditions can be utterly exhausting.

As with any anxiety related condition one finds soon they are forced to enter the complex health arena of *'chicken and the egg'*. What comes first? The anxiety or the anxiety related condition? Answers on a postcard!

Certainly, the one thing *every* client with vertigo, tinnitus or labyrinthitis seems to have in common is a fairly defined *fixation* about their symptoms. The vertigo client becomes as frightened of the potential spinning episodes in a similar manner to the way the panic attack client becomes frightened of the *randomness* of their attacks. These clients feel, understandably so, completely out of control, and that mindset can further promote an emotional state of fear and anxiety. In TCM, certainly, fear is believed to *eat up* the vital life energy residing in the kidney, which in turn is linked to the ears.

Encouragingly, during a reflexology session the tinnitus client will often report the ringing or buzzing has dissipated, and a verbal acknowledgment of this can certainly support the suggestion that more instances of focused relaxation might be equally beneficial. Many clients, when offered the TCM context, will often go on to acknowledge a natural tendency towards anxious thinking, as well as admitting to feelings of physical and emotional exhaustion. Similarly, the vertigo or labyrinthitis client often also benefits from information and a new *context* in which to consider their condition.

Certainly, the key words to highlight with this particular with this client group would be *rest*, *physical strength building*, and *focused relaxation*. Finally, this is, without a doubt, one of the client groups where therapeutic change is far more likely to manifest when the client and practitioner work together.

The Client

Karen is a 56 year old married mother of three grown up children, and in full time employment. Karen has suffered from short periods of vertigo throughout her adult life, and at the first session reported she was deep in the midst of a worsening, four month long acute phase, and struggling to cope. Karen's GP, whilst entirely sympathetic, has been unable to offer any defining solution, and so armed with a friends recommendation, Karen decided to try reflexology.

During the initial consultation Karen was able to talk about the dynamics of her family life, revealing she had recently condensed her full time job to a four day week, in order to free up time to help with her grand-daughters childcare. Karen also talked about how she'd raised her three children alone, and felt an enormous sense of responsibility during her younger years, and revealed that today, even though life is easier in many ways, she can still find it difficult to allow her internal sense of responsibility slide. Karen was additionally able to identify she finds it difficult to quiet the constant narrative (chit chat) in her mind. She remarked she *thinks* constantly, makes endless lists of jobs to be done, and finds it hard to sit down and relax; always feeling there is more to be done. Finally, Karen was able express how frightened she now felt that the condition would never go away. Karen attended for reflexology across eight weeks. During this time Karen made changes in her personal life and made more time for her own needs. By the seventh session Karen's symptoms had all but receded completely, and Karen was feeling more able accept the concept of relaxation into her life.

The Sessions

- I was able to educate Karen about the hypothalamus-pituitary-adrenal axis, and let her know how feelings of stress and stress hormones are able to affect her wider body.

- I was able to give Karen a context for the spells of vertigo by explaining the basic principles of TCM (kidney-bladder-ear-fear & fright), and explain that vertigo might be viewed as an exhaustion condition, according to TCM.

- I was able to teach Karen a simple mindful deep breathing technique to support calm in her mind.

- I was able to talk to Karen about self care and help her to form a plan simplifying the coming week and providing space for more instances of self care.

- I was able to listen and authenticate Karen's experiences.

- I was able to touch, educate, and offer support.

Summary

I cannot offer the reader any *evidence* as to why reflexology might impact so positively with this particular client group, given the right conditions. Perhaps, because of increased periods of deep relaxation the brains plasticity is permitting some form of neural modification of the auditory or proprioception system? A reboot if you will? Perhaps this is the brains natural reaction to any form of disturbance, but in some cases fear and distress become an obstacle?

Perhaps, these conditions are more generally associated with the autoimmune system; the condition perpetually compounded by elevated states of accompanying anxiety? In either scenario, the brain seems to wholly approve of reflexology, and the modality seems able to provide the space for some form of re-balance to occur.

Karen told me about the vertigo during our telephone consultation. Based on my previous experience and existing base knowledge I almost immediately associate this type of condition to a state of physical and emotional exhaustion; defined more specifically as excessive, long term cognitive activity, feelings of anxiety, and probable long term activation of the HPA axis. Up to this point however *(and this bit is really important)*, everything I *think* I know is merely my assumption.

Part of my role as a therapist is to present information to my clients and explore any obvious possibilities. It is the client however who must decide if the offered context fits within their own experience. If as therapists we hope to engage our clients in more frequent states of autonomy and self directed change, then it is crucial, *particularly with anxious clients*, a new context in which to appreciate *why* more instance of self care and focused periods of relaxation are recommended is offered. The client must also learn to take care of themselves outside of the weekly sessions.

I wonder how long it had been since Karen focused upon her own personal needs? Together, we spent eight sessions of 60 minutes focused entirely on Karen's experiences and considering her own unique requirements. I wonder also if Karen has ever been quite so educated about the delicate and intimate relationship between her emotions, her brain, and her physical body?

Knowledge can be a powerful tool when used to invoke autonomy and client directed change.

Isn't it amazing what a good cut of time, some delicious human touch, a dash of clinical knowledge, a sprinkling of Chinese folklore, and a healthy dose of care can do?

That is mind, body, spirit.

Relational Reflexology

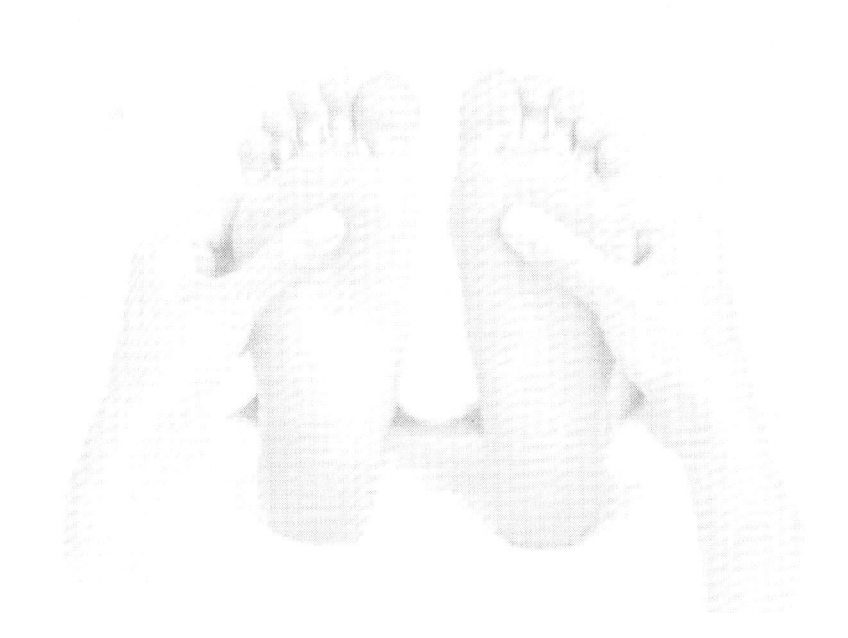

Clinical Information Relating to Sub-Fertility

Conception and Early Pregnancy

Fertilisation

Fertilisation can be defined as the joining of a sperm (gamete) and a mature egg (ovum). It is estimated only 100/4million sperm reach the typical fertilisation site, the fallopian tubes. To penetrate the egg the sperm must break through two barriers surrounding the ovum; the corona radiata and the zona pellucida. On reaching the plasma membrane of the egg a reaction is initiated which prevents further sperm from breaking through to the egg membrane.

Once inside the sperm sheds its tail and the two nuclei (23 chromosomes from the sperm and 23 chromosomes from the ovum) fuse and develop into a zygote. The chromosomes carry the generic information required as the building blocks of life. The sex of a baby is determined by male gametes because female ovum carry only X sex chromosomes, whilst sperm carries both X or Y sex chromosomes.

Pre-Embryonic Period

The zygote begins a process of dividing by mitosis until it reaches 16 cells referred to as a morula. The morula begins to fills with fluid and the cells form two separate groups, now called a blastocyst. The embryoblast makes up the inner layer of cells developing into the foetus, whilst the outer layer is called a trophoblast and develops into part of the placenta.

Once in contact with the thickened endometrium the trophoblast utilises specialised cells designed to spread and grown into the endometrium and assist implantation.

Implantation

The blastocyst secretes hCG hormone to maintain the corpus luteum which in turn secretes progesterone, maintaining the endometrial lining of the uterus and helping to ensure the blastocyst remains embedded within the endometrium.

As the placenta begins to form it takes responsibility for producing progesterone. The embryoblast within the blastocyst forms 3 primary germ layers; the ectoderm, mesoderm, and endoderm. The ectoderm forms the epidermis of skin, hair, nails, sweat glands, tooth enamel, lining of oral cavity, anal cavity and vagina, brain, sensory organs, lens of eye and epithelium of conjunctiva, pituitary gland and adrenal medulla.

The mesoderm forms the kidneys, blood vessels, muscle tissues, connective tissue, adrenal cortex and reproductive organs. The endoderm forms the digestive tract, lungs, tonsils, liver, pancreas, thyroid, parathyroid, anterior pituitary and thymus glands and urogenital systems.

Formation of the Placenta and Amniotic Fluid

The formation of foetal and maternal tissue makes the functional unit called the placenta. The placenta allows for nutrients and waste products to diffuse between the foetal blood system and that of the mother. The amnion is a membranous attached to the placenta which fills with water (amniotic fluid) around two weeks after fertilisation and provides protection and buoyancy for the developing embryo.

The amniotic fluid eventually contains vital nutrients which aid in the growth of the foetus and in the later stages of pregnancy the amniotic fluid is utilised to prepare the digestive organs for function (swallowing the fluid), and with lung development (breathing the fluid in).

For most women the first sign of pregnancy is a missed period (menses). This occurs because the blastocyst triggers the release of hCG (human chorionic gonadotropin) the hormone recognised by pregnancy tests. Human pregnancy lasts approximately 40 weeks. The medical term for a developing baby is embryo (early weeks) and from then onwards, until birth, a foetus.

Sub-Fertility – A Definition

Experts believe the chance of spontaneous conception occurring in the first month of active trying lies at around 30%. Thereafter the chance falls to around 5% by the end of the first active year. Sub-fertility is defined as failure to conceive after one year of regular sexual intercourse.

A natural reduction in fertility occurs in women in their late 30s and early 40s, with the chance of conceiving for women between 35-39 years half that of women aged 19-26. Genetic defects found in older sperm and oocytes (immature ovum) are thought to impair gamete (sperm) function and embryonic development.

Sub-fertility can be clinically defined as:

- **Primary** sub-fertility: a delay for couples with no previous pregnancies.
- **Secondary** sub-fertility: a delay for a couple who have previously conceived; but the pregnancy may not have been successful (ectopic pregnancy or miscarriage).

Research has demonstrated that the ovulatory cycle lasts approximately six days, with optimum levels peaking 2 days before ovulation, and dipping by the day of ovulation. The chance of conception is therefore increased if sperm is deposited into the genital tract before ovulation.

Experts also believe BMI (body mass index) impacts on sub-fertility with research demonstrating women are more likely to achieve conception with a BMI of >20 <30. Smoking, caffeine and recreational drugs are also believed to reduce the chance of natural conception. Whilst it is difficult for researchers to ascertain the precise effects of smoking it has been estimated for example that smokers are 3.4 times more likely to take 12 months or more to conceive. Researchers also believe increased sub-fertility rates may be associated with factors such as a rise in environmental oestrogenic pollutants; correlating with a recent decline in sperm counts in Europe and North America.

Clinical Conditions Relating to Sub-Fertility

Sub-fertility issues can be broadly categorised as disorders relating to ovulation, tubal damage, unexplained, male factors and other hormonally related conditions such as endometriosis.

Amenorrhea

The generic term used to refer to the absence of a woman's menstrual period. Amenorrhea is not a disease, rather it is the generic name given simply to the symptom of absent menstruation. Secondary amenorrhea is more common and refers to either the temporary or permanent ending of periods in a woman who has menstruated normally in the past. Many women miss a period occasionally however amenorrhea only clinically occurs if a woman misses three or more periods in succession.

Primary amenorrhea is a rare occurrence in a therapist's private practice as it relates specifically to the failure to start to menstruate by the age of 16. It can sometimes be difficult to find the cause of amenorrhea. The GP will often perform blood tests to check for signs of androgen excess, oestrogen deficiency or other problems associated with the endocrine system such as thyroid disorders. Typical causes of secondary amenorrhea might include:

- excessive weight loss such as that which occurs as a result of anorexia nervosa or bulimia

- excessive weight gain or general poor diet

- emotional stress or depression

- stopping birth control

- strenuous physical exercise

- hypothyroidism

- PCOS (Poly Cystic Ovarian Syndrome)

Anovulation

Ovulation disorders occur in around 30% of women experiencing sub-fertility problems and often present with irregular periods (oligomenorrhoea) or an absence of periods (amenorrhea).

PCOS (Polycystic Ovarian Syndrome)

Polycystic ovary syndrome (PCOS) is an increasingly common female endocrine disorder in women of reproductive age and believed to be one of the leading causes of sub-fertility in the West. As well as menstrual difficulties women with PCOS also experience high levels of androgens (masculinising hormones) in the body.

Symptoms can display as adult acne, hirsutism (hair growth), androgynous alopecia (hair loss), lethargy, depression and sub-fertility. There is also a strong link between PCOS and insulin resistance, further linked to a tendency in these women towards weight gain, central obesity and type II diabetes, which can in turn increase the chance of developing anovulation.

Clinical Diagnosis and Treatment for PCOS

Not all women with PCOS however have polycystic ovaries (PCO), nor do all women with ovarian cysts have PCOS, and so the symptoms and severity of the syndrome vary greatly among affected women. A clinical diagnosis of PCOS is normally made in a woman experiencing anovulation via blood tests to confirm excessive androgen levels, and to check on the concentrations of luteinising hormone, follicle stimulating hormone and estradiol. Additionally, a vaginal ultrasound exam of the pelvis can be carried out to confirm the presence of cysts.

In the first instance women with PCOS are advised to lose weight where necessary. One front-line medical treatment utilised to treat PCOS is an insulin sensitising medication called Metformin which acts to support the pancreas (the organ which secretes the hormone insulin). Once insulin resistance in the body is corrected and rebalanced the endocrine system in general seems to stabilise and ovulation and the menstrual cycle often spontaneously restart. Symptomatic treatments of PCOS might include the use of anti-androgens, and/or steroid hormones such as the oral contraceptive. Relating to the treatment of PCOS related sub-fertility the use of chomiphene citrate is often considered to induce ovulation, in addition to IVF depending on the age of the woman.

Tubal Sub-Fertility

Fallopian tubes are highly specialised organs responsible for picking up and transporting eggs, sperm and embryos. Eggs are fertilised in the Fallopian tube and the first stages of embryo development occur in the tubes.

Scar tissue present in the fallopian tubes occurring as a result of historic PID (pelvic inflammatory disease) can hinder egg pickup and transport, fertilisation and then transportation of the embryo to the uterus. Endometriosis can also leave scar tissue, as can previous pelvic surgery. Fallopian tubes can be lost entirely as a result of tubal ectopic pregnancy, which is also more common in women with scarred fallopian tubes. In many cases of tubal sub-fertility women are referred directly for IVF after a clinical diagnosis.

Dysmenorrhea

Dysmenorrhea is not a disease, rather it is the generic name given to excessive menstrual pain which has a tendency to interfere with normal daily routines and activities. Dysmenorrhea can often co-exist with heavy menstrual bleeding, known as Menorrhagia.

Primary dysmenorrhea is menstrual pain in otherwise healthy women normally occurring from the onset of menstruation and where no other underlying medical condition is present.

Secondary dysmenorrhea is menstrual pain which develops later in women who had normal menstrual cycles and is often related with medical conditions affecting the uterus or pelvis.

The GP may perform blood tests or refer the patient for an exploratory laparoscopy or pelvic scan. Typical causes of secondary dysmenorrhea might include endometriosis, ovarian cysts, uterine fibroids, pelvic inflammatory disease, copper IUD.

Endometriosis

Endometriosis is a medical condition in which cells from the lining of the uterus (endometrium) appear and grow outside of the uterine cavity and present in 20-40% of women who present with sub-fertility problems. The endometrial cells react to hormonal changes and behave in a similar manner to cells found inside the uterus. The most common areas for these cells to found are in the fallopian tubes, ovaries, bladder, bowel, vagina or rectum. Endometriosis is often a chronic condition which causes painful and/or heavy menstrual periods. The condition can also be responsible for severe pelvic, abdominal and lower back pain as well as a lack of energy, and in severe cases depression and fertility problems. Some women however suffer few or no symptoms at all and a diagnosis might only be made as a result of deeper investigation such as a laparoscopy.

The cause of endometriosis is not fully known. The most common theory is that cells from the womb lining (endometrium) do not leave the body properly during the menstrual cycle and instead embed onto the organs of the pelvis. Each month because the endometrial cells behave in the same way as those that line the uterus, they go through the same process of thickening and shedding, and his can lead to pain, swelling and even damage to the fallopian tubes or ovaries (known as endometriotic lesions). Complications resulting from endometriosis can include internal scarring, adhesions, pelvic and ovarian cysts, bowel obstruction and pelvic adhesions. Infertility can often be related to scar tissue and anatomical distortions caused by the endometrial cells, however it is believed that endometriosis may also interfere in more subtle ways, specifically that endometrial lesions may release other factors (inflammatory cytokines, and other chemical agents) that may further interfere with reproduction.

Clinical Diagnosis and Treatment for Endometriosis

- **Laparoscopy**: a commonly used keyhole surgery procedure used to diagnose endometriosis.

- **Topical Analgesia**: Non-steroid anti-inflammatory drugs (NSAID), such as ibuprofen or codeine, are often used to treat the pain associated with endometriosis, principally because they act against the inflammation (swelling) caused by endometriosis, as well as helping to ease pain and discomfort.

- **Hormones**: The aim of hormone treatments (GnRH) is to limit or stop the production of oestrogen in the body and therefore reduce any stimulating effect oestrogen has on the growth of the endometrial tissue. Hormone treatments however have no effect on endometrial lesions and do little to improve fertility.

- **Surgery**: A laparoscopy is a commonly used keyhole surgery procedure used to diagnose and treat endometriosis and related ovarian cysts. All grades of endometriosis can be successfully treated with this minimally invasive technique. Heat, lasers or an electric current are applied to destroy the affected tissue.

- A **laparotomy** is a less common major surgery only used if the endometriosis is severe and extensive. Although both types of surgery can often relieve symptoms temporarily it is not uncommon for symptoms to recur, particularly if some endometrial cell tissue is left behind during surgery, and for this reason it is not uncommon for women suffering from severe endometriosis to undergo several laparoscopies across her fertile years.

Fibroids

Fibroids are benign tumours of the myometrium and occur in 30% of women are are estimated to have a detrimental effect of fertility in up to 10% of women. Fibroids can be reduced in size temporarily by hormonal medications, such as gonodatrophin releasing analogues (GnRH), however once re-exposed to a more oestrogen rich environment they often start to grow again. Surgical removal of larger fibroids is often carried out after a period of shrinking brought about through the administration of GnRH medication.

Unexplained/Non-Specific Sub-Fertility

Whilst unexplained infertility is not a medically diagnosed condition in the traditional sense it does encompass a large percentage of women who present for supportive reflexology experiencing sub-fertility, and the group is thought to account for up to 25% of women who present for investigation is specialist fertility units. Often the most frustrating diagnosis for women, a hypothesis pertaining to the 'hospitable womb' might well go some way to better explaining this large group of women.

Repeated Miscarriage

It has been estimated that miscarriage occurs in 15-20% of all pregnancies, usually in the first three months. After a woman experiences three or more miscarriages, it's referred to clinically as 'repeated miscarriage'. The causes of miscarriage are varied:

- **Chromosomal**: one of the most common causes of miscarriage, thought to comprise of over 50% of all miscarriages. Potentially, the number of chromosomes in the foetus, the structure of the chromosome, or even the genetic material that they carry may present a problem.

- **Abnormalities of the uterus** such as a double uterus and conditions such as fibroids can sometimes cause problems.

- **Hormonal imbalance**

- **Immunity problems**: sometimes the body can view the foetus as a foreign body and so attacks the pregnancy. Blood tests can sometimes determine if a woman has this immunity problem.

Male Sub-Fertility

Sub-fertility is thought to affect one in 20 men. The results of two sperm samples are normally analysed by the GP around 6 weeks apart. Male clinical sub-fertility terminology includes:

- **Oligozoospermia** - Reduced number of sperm

- **Asthenozoospermia** – Reduced sperm motility

- **Teratozoospermia** – Increased abnormal morphology in sperm

- **Azoospermia** – Absence of sperm

- **Necrozoospermia** – All sperm non-viable or non-motile

- **Oligooasthenoteratozoospermia** (sperm variable all abnormal) is the most common cause of male sub-fertility with male sub-fertility rarely caused by hormonal imbalances; rather lifestyle and environmental factors are thought to impact more directly. In the first instance men are encouraged to make lifestyle changes where appropriate. For most couples where male sub-fertility is indicated however assisted conception techniques can offer a good chance of conception.

A **normal** range sperm sample demonstrates:

- 2ml volume & sperm concentration of >2 million/ml.

- Motility > 50% progressive or 25% rapidly progressive

- Morphology >15% normal forms

- White blood cells <1 million/ml

- Immunobead or mixed anti-globulin reaction test <50% (presence of antibodies coating the sperm)

Clinical and Medical Intervention

Primary (GP) protocols relating to **female** sub-fertility can include:

- Cervical smear

- Test for chlamydia and other STDs

- Ovulation testing: checks progesterone levels seven days before menstruation

- Blood tests to determine hormone levels: including TSH (thyroid stimulating hormone); FSH (follicle stimulating hormone); LH (luteinising hormone) and estradiol levels. FHS and LH tests are generally carried out between day 2 and 6 of the menstrual cycle. These tests can potentially also rule out early menopause.

- Referral to a gynaecological unit or in some cases directly to a specialist IVF unit.

For **men** (GP):

- Sperm test checking morphology (shape), motility (movement) and count
- Test for Chlamydia

Common **secondary** protocols for sub-fertility include referral to a consultant gynaecologist or specialist fertility unit for:

- A **laparoscopic investigation** is a commonly used keyhole surgery procedure used to investigate, diagnose (and treat) pelvic abnormalities and clinical conditions such as endometriosis.

- **Clomifene Citrate** is a fertility drug used to stimulate and/or regulate ovulation by blocking oestrogen receptors in the pituitary gland, leading to increased production of FSH. Increased FHS levels in turn stimulate the development of dominant ovarian follicles. Generally clomifene is only prescribed within specialist fertility units because of an additional requirement for uterine ultrasound monitoring; linked to a risk of multiple follicle development and in some cases hyper stimulation of the ovaries.

- **Intrauterine Insemination (IUI)** washes and separates fast moving healthy sperm, returning it to the woman's uterus at the time of ovulation, via the use of a catheter. IUI might be performed stimulated or un-stimulated. When the cycle is stimulated the woman is also given fertility drugs to better ensure ovulation occurs. The success rate of IUI is only slightly higher than that of natural conception.

- **In Vitro Fertilisation (IVF):** IVF involves gathering oocytes (obtained surgically) from ovarian follicles and prepared sperm which are then fertilised outside the body (in vitro means in glass). Embryos derived from these oocytes are then re-implanted in the woman's uterus.

IVF (In Vitro Fertilisation)

Information is provided here relating to a generic IVF protocol. In reality however, each specialist fertility unit has its own individual way of carrying out the protocol. Some units might start on a particular day of the woman's menstrual cycle, some don't. Some units might administer antibiotics to the women and her partner prior to commencing the protocol, again some don't. Some units might use a nasal spray to down regulate the women during the first phase, whilst some might use a pen-injection. Some doctors will 'tweak' the IVF drugs to suit the individual woman; whilst some units may have a one protocol fits all policy. Increasingly units are providing short-protocol IVF, over in less than three weeks. Given the nature of the specialism the IVF protocol is not carried out in every local hospital, and so many reflexology practitioners may only be within range of one or two specialist IVF units. It is essential practitioners gather research regarding their local unit/s individual clinic protocols.

In Vitro Fertilisation (IVF) for women involves:

- **Step 1**: the down-regulation phase. Women administer drugs daily/twice daily (usually GnRH) to suppress pituitary function.mTreatment is administered via a nasal spray or a daily injection. Down regulation is principally used in super ovulation regimens to prevent the surge of luteinising hormone and the release of oocytes prematurely.

- **Step 2**: stimulating egg supply. Once the menstrual cycle is successfully suppressed, FSH (follicle stimulating hormone) is administered by injection for approximately 12 days.

- **Step 3**: monitoring. Vaginal ultrasound scans are performed regularly (particularly in the final week of the drug protocol) in order to ensure the woman is responding to the drugs correctly. When the follicles measure a sufficient size (> 18mm in diameter) women are given the go ahead to administer an injection of human chorionic gonadotrophin which helps eggs to mature and occurs around 34-38 hours prior to egg collection

- **Step 4**: egg collection. Eggs are usually collected by ultrasound guidance, with the woman under sedation.

- **Step 5**: insemination, fertilisation and embryo transfer. Eggs and sperm are mixed and cultured by the embryologist for approximately 16–20 hours. Fertilised embryos are allowed to develop for a further 24-48 hours, before the best embryo(s) are chosen for transfer back to the woman's uterus (normally one or two embryos are returned: numbers are restricted by guidelines because of the risks associated with multiple births). Embryos have usually developed by this stage into four, six or eight cells respectively. In some cases embryos are allowed to develop to blasocyst stage (day 5). Women are required to administer progesterone medication (normally pessaries) for a minimum of two weeks to help ensure the lining of the uterus remains in place.

IVF for men

- **Sperm collection**. A fresh sample of sperm is retrieved generally at the time of egg collection (unless frozen sperm is being used) and the healthiest sperm then selected for the IVF/ICSI process.

Intra-Cytoplasmic Sperm Injection (ICSI)

An **ICSI** protocol for a woman is exactly the same as the IVF protocol. The difference lies in the manner in which the egg is inseminated and fertilised. ICSI is a specialist variant of IVF where the embryologist injects a single sperm directly into the cytoplasm of the egg. ICSI is generally carried out when there is a problem with the sperm. This might be connected to poor count, morphology or motility, or it might be as a result of sperm collected post vasectomy, or because sperm has been previously frozen or gathered surgically from the epididymis or testes.

Frozen Embryo Transfer

Additional embryos cultivated by IVF, measured to be of sufficient quality may be suitable for freezing depending on the individual facilities available to each IVF unit, and their associated protocols. Shortened IVF protocols are common place in instances where there are frozen viable embryo's available. Interesting research has demonstrated that the success rates for frozen embryo transfers in IVF patients may be higher than success rates with convention IVF protocols.

Short Protocol IVF (Soft IVF)

Short protocol IVF cycles were previously utilised with older women who perhaps displayed lower egg stocks, or who had not responded well to a previous IVF protocol. Short protocol IVF is now increasingly also being used with younger women.

Relational Reflexology

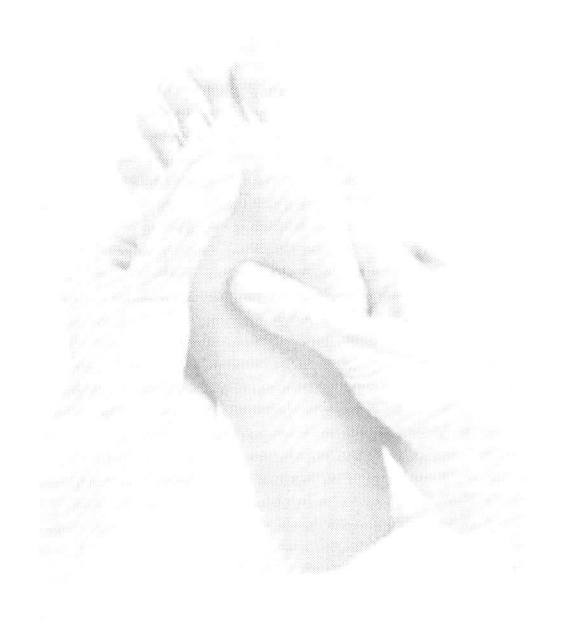

The Emotional Impact of Sub-Fertility

"Everywhere I go I feel like I'm being stalked by pregnant women. It just seems so unfair."

- A reflexology client

The statement above is fairly representative of the feelings of many women who enter a reflexology practitioner's therapy room looking for support with sub-fertility. The statement perhaps best reflects the duality of a woman's experience emotionally. Initially we're drawn to almost a fixation with pregnancy; to the extent that everywhere the woman turns she can see pregnancy in others. The second part of the statement perhaps simply expresses the deep sadness and grief like feelings often experienced by these women. Indeed grief, sadness, anger, frustration, anxiety and fear are all familiar emotions for the sub-fertility client.

Women sometimes talk of their deep sadness when friends become pregnant, and then their later feelings of shame because they know deep inside they feel envious. Some women find the sight of a pregnant woman difficult to endure, whilst for others it is the sight of a mother pushing her pram. Siblings, relations, friends, workmates and even hardly known acquaintances all seem to be able to pro-create easily enough, without assistance, and irritatingly some even go on to do it twice! Women come to know their bodies intimately, charting basal temperatures and testing for ovulation, yet often lose faith in their bodies completely.

Women recount tails of engaging robotically with their partners and husbands, and talk of how fertility problems have damaged their sex life and feelings of intimacy and closeness. The dreaded arrival of the menstrual bleed is simply a reminder of how they've failed yet again, each month, each failure only adding to a deep sub-conscious fear that they will never become pregnant. Women dealing with sub-fertility can exist in a state of pretending to be happy on the surface, whilst experiencing deep pain on the inside. Friends and family smile supportively and make noises of optimism and bright futures. Comments like 'you just need to relax' or 'have a holiday' are well meant and common place, yet all the while the women alone with their fears are screaming inside, tortured by a never-ending longing to have a baby. It might take the average women between two and three years of trying to conceive naturally before she is referred to a specialist unit. The sub-fertility journey can take an enormous toll both physically and emotionally.

The Emotional Impact of IVF

It is important to remember that for most women undergoing IVF being referred to a specialist fertility unit is but the latest stop on a very long journey. Initially, most women feel only relief when an IVF referral letter arrives, finally they will see the doctors who really know what they're doing! Finally arrives the day of the first appointment, and no matter how well trained and welcoming the staff are, no matter how inviting the environment of the IVF unit, the moment a woman is given the date schedule for her IVF protocol and she becomes aware of what lies ahead of her, fear and panic can often set in.

No matter how astonishing the science of IVF might be the reality of the protocol for most women might be best described as negotiating a path of hurdles. One cannot move forward to the next phase of treatment until X, Y or Z has been achieved, and at all times there is a worry the protocol might be abandoned if the woman does not respond accordingly. If the protocol is completed through to the egg collection phase, attention turns to the concern over how many eggs will be retrieved successfully, of those eggs how many will fertilise successfully, and will they be good enough grade embryos? Post embryo transfer a woman waits and tries hard not to agonise over the next ten days until either a menstrual bleed occurs spontaneously, or a test confirms either a pregnancy or a failed cycle. It is easy to imagine how a woman might find this entire process deeply distressing.

Women's Words on Sub-Fertility

- "I thought (pregnancy) would never happen"

- "I am alone in it all"

- "Constant bleeding and hormonal irregularity meant my body felt completely alien to me"

- "I'd become a shadow of the person I used to be"

- "You try to remain positive and happy but it hurts, and you start to wonder what you've done wrong to deserve such a harsh punishment"

- "After 3 unsuccessful IVF attempts we were left devastated"

- "Every advert seems to be baby stuff; every soap (on TV) has an unwanted pregnancy story!"

- "Hubby tries to be supportive but each month when I get upset he tells me 'I told you not to get your hopes up!' How can you remain positive and upbeat and not hope each month?"

- "I felt it was all my fault"

- "Simple day to day tasks were crushing. Walking round the supermarket through aisles of babies in prams, or expectant mothers tenderly rubbing their growing bumps made me want to stay at home and hide from the world" "Everything seemed to come back to one thought; will I have another baby?"

- "I realised how stressed and deflated I had become as a result of the repeated failures"

Summary

It would clearly be entirely unprofessional to attempt any form of therapeutic work with this vulnerable client group without first gaining a deeper respect and appreciation of how sub-fertility issues can impact across the lives of women.

The sub-fertility journey can be hugely disempowering. A journey in which a woman can lose both connection and trust with her body and with hope and her future – both mind and body equally challenged.

Reflexology and the Whole Person Sub-Fertility

"Reproduction is one of the strongest of biological reflexes – just ask a salmon leaping upstream to spawn or male of various species risking life and limb for access to females, or any adolescent with that crazed steroid look. But when it comes to the pirouettes and filigrees of sexuality, stress can wreak havoc with subtleties."

- Robert Sapolsky

The Hospitable Womb

When considering the potential emotional and physical challenges faced by many individuals it might be easy to imagine why, in this particular client group, the fight or flight response might be on high alert. How might the body feel about the possibility of nurturing new life when deep in the brain the perception is processed as if the individual was being chased by a hungry lion or a similar type threat?

The fear response makes no comparison between real and perceived fear - to the hypothalamus a bad tempered boss at work feels much the same as a hungry lion, and it *will* react accordingly. Carl Rogers, the well know humanistic psychologist, proposed the existence of a self–actualising tendency. The self actualising tendency dictates all life possesses an innate drive to become *everything* it can possibly can be; to achieve its full potential. Self-actualising modern day human beings have learned to manipulate a woman's body into believing it is in a state of menopause, only then to be stimulated in the opposite direction to such a degree that multiple follicles and eggs are produced in the ovaries. That particular feat is balanced alongside assuring the lining of the womb develops sufficiently to host a returned fertilised embryo.

Eggs are collected from ovaries microscopically and sparked into life by an embryologist using a microscope and a glass dish, before being returned to a woman's uterus. The IVF process is undoubtedly an astonishing scientific feat and a credit to the enquiring human mind. We are indeed fortunate to live in a society where such specialised clinical work is valued.

A woman's inner drive to experience pregnancy and motherhood is absolutely deserving of such time, research and financial investment, and there are many women today feel a huge debt of gratitude to specialist IVF and fertility units. The writer is confident however even the most experienced consultants engaged in the field of IVF still scratch their heads from time to time and wonder why it is, even when top grade embryos are returned into a perfectly lined uterus, the generic success rate of IVF is around 26%? (HFEA 2009).

Research demonstrates success rates for frozen embryo transfers might be higher than those linked to conventional IVF protocols. It might be useful to reflect on the emotional mind-set of a woman who already knows she has potentially viable embryos available for transfer. How might this prior knowledge alter a women's perception of her chances of success?

Women in under-developed countries often live in poor conditions with little food, poor sanitation and little or no medical support. One thing is almost certain though. There are generally lots of babies around! What is perceived in the West as an intensely stressful lifestyle is often, sadly, but the norm for these women. Could this frame of reference be dictating a more *normally* functioning HPA response? Admittedly, we have the privilege of clean running water and central heating here in the West, but our stressful lifestyles and constant requirement to be ever productive and busy may well be leading us to disrespect some of the innate autonomic systems deep within our brains. Systems designed by nature above all else to keep us safe.

"The fight of flight alarm reaction exists today for the same purpose evolution originally assigned to it; to enable us to survive. What has happened is that we have lost touch with the gut feeling designed to be out warning systems." (Mate, 2003)

The self actualising tendency draws attention to the concept that life, given appropriate conditions to flourish, will often find a way to do so. Perhaps this concept might also be considered when attempting to appreciate why increasing numbers of women in the West are being diagnosed with non-specific sub-fertility, and how this concept might also be impacting on IVF success rates? After all, there are many animals on our planet instinctively drawn to finding a safe place to nest before pro-creation occurs. Why would human beings be any different? The concept of stress in our modern world has become somewhat blurred, and its consequences morphed to such a degree that dealing well with stress has almost become a badge of honour - viewed as a sign of advanced coping mechanisms and an ability to successfully juggle all of life's complicated demands. In reality, the principles of human homeostasis demonstrate quite clearly that for every *effect* there also exists a *counter effect*. Where high and sustained levels of stress exist in the human individual, so too can perturbations of the wider endocrine system.

The concept of adopting a professional rationale for practice is important for modern day professional reflexology practitioners. Any rationale for practice should ideally strive to encompass both the individual practitioner's theoretical stance of practice, as well as focusing upon developing a better understanding of each presenting client group, or specific health condition. With regards to supporting the generic sub-fertility group a valid rationale for practice can certainly be constructed through leaning upon existing clinical and academic research. Specifically that where examination focused upon:

- The effects of real or perceived stress on human health and sub-fertility.
- The effects of reflexology on stress and anxiety.

- The effects of interpersonal touch.

- The potential impact of the therapeutic (reflexology) relationship.

- Existential benefit stemming from increased client autonomy and self-directed change.

Stress and Pregnancy

Studies examining the influences of psychoneuroendocrine processes on women's health and foetal development have demonstrated both cardiovascular and neuroendocrine responses to stressors are attenuated during human pregnancy, and that increased cardiovascular reactivity is associated with:

"shorter gestation, lower birth weight, increased risk of preeclampia and vulnerability for postpartum depression." (Christian, 2012).

Other researchers (Wadhwa, 2005) believe maternal stress responses may indeed have life-long effects on off-spring health and that;

"maternal environment exerts significant influence on foetal neurodevelopment processes related to recognition, memory and habituation".

Culhane et al, (2001), looking at the influence of maternal psychosocial stress on the development of reproductive tract infections amongst a large group of socially disadvantaged women found that:

"stress related endocrine processes modulate immune function in the context of reproductive tract infection and inflammation".

Studies have also demonstrated that interventions such as guided imagery, yoga and relaxation (DiPietro et al, 2011); (Urich et al, 1991); (Beddoe et al, 2009); (Beddoe & Lee, 2008) can be effective in reducing maternal heart rate and subjective feelings of stress.

Stress and Sub-Fertility

In normally responding individuals the brain releases GnRH (gonadotrophin releasing hormone), which stimulates the pituitary to release LH (luteinizing hormone) and FHS (follicle stimulating hormone). Luteinizing hormone stimulates the ovaries to synthesise estrogen and the testes to release testosterone.

The activation of FSH in women stimulates the ovaries to release eggs, and in men stimulates sperm production. Stress has been demonstrated to elevate levels of adrenocorticotropic hormone (ACTH) and cortisol in the blood and researchers believe these increases may:

"At least temporarily amplify the effects of the pituitary-adrenal axis on other tissues." (Daruna, 2012).

Because the hypothalamus is in two-way communication with the brain centre that process emotions:

"It is through the HPA axis that emotions exert their most direct effects on the immune system and on other organs." (Mate, 2003)

Indeed stress has been demonstrated as activating the hypothalmic-pituitary-adrenal (HPA) axis in turn inhibits gonadotrophin-releasing hormone (Gn-RH) release, possibly through the effects of opioid peptides.

Inhibition of Gn-RH release leads to decreased luteinizing hormone (LH) and follicle-stimulating hormone (FSH) levels in the circulation and ultimately reduced estradiol in females and testosterone in males:

"Thus psychosocial stress appears to cause the decrease of gonadal steroids." (Daruna, 2012)

The HPA axis and the reproductive system demonstrate a complex relationship. CRH and cortisol receptors are;

"abundant in the endometrium, myometrium, and the ovaries." (Demyttenaere et al, 1994)

Stress can also inhibit progesterone levels which can in turn disrupt the maturation of uterine walls. The release of prolactin during times of stress can further interfere with the activity of progesterone, making any fertilised egg:

"Much less likely to implant normally." (Sapolsky, 2004)

A study published in the 'Canadian Journal of Diagnosis' (Prior, 1997) found that:

"Subtle hormonal disruption can even occur amongst women who report regular periods and no symptoms",

The study also demonstrated anovulation problems in women:

"Are caused by adaptations to life cycle, changes in weight, psychosocial stresses, excessive exercise or illness."

Indeed experts believe the hormones related to female reproduction to be:

"Exquisitely sensitive to women's psychological states and to the stresses in their lives." (Mate, 2003).

Stress and IVF

One of the main difficulties in evaluating the success rate of IVF is establishing the particular factors which make a real difference. Experts such as Robert Sapolsky (2004), a professor of biology and neurology at Stanford University, believe the *'stressfulness'* of IVF procedures contribute to the low success rates.

Interestingly, IVF patients with functional disorders of the HPA axis often demonstrate higher stress-scores than women where sub-fertility is associated with anatomical problems (tube obstruction, malformations of the reproductive organs). It has also been demonstrated that stress and anxiety are very common in sub-fertility patients, especially those undergoing IVF (Salvatore et al., 2001). Some IVF studies have demonstrated that the chance to conceive and to bring the pregnancy to a good end is smaller if the patient reports more stress or anxiety at the onset of therapy (Demyttenaere et al., 1994).

In 2008 Manheimer et al., (2008) reviewed the effect of acupuncture on IVF, comparing the results of seven different trials, including 1366 women. Results overall demonstrate the application of acupuncture immediately before and after embryo transfer improves rates of pregnancy and live birth among women undergoing IVF. Another small research study (Balk et al., 2009) specifically looked at the relationship between perceived stress, acupuncture, and pregnancy in IVF patients. In this study the mechanism of acupuncture was not specifically studied. Rather the research attempted to establish if *perceived* stress factored in IVF success rates. The study utilised a 10-item stress questionnaire to establish patients stress levels before and during embryo transfer; concluding;

"The acupuncture regimen was associated with less stress both before and after embryo transfer and it possibly improved pregnancy rates. Lower perceived stress at the time of embryo transfer may play a role in an improved pregnancy rate".

Given the proven effects of persistent and acute stress on both foetal development and maternal health, it makes complete sense that complex systems in the body might trigger a biological defense mechanism designed to prevent conception occurring in the first instance. A defense mechanism ultimately designed to protect life energy of the host organism - the mother.

Sub-Fertility and Traditional Chinese Medicine

The spleen, liver and kidneys energies are considered important according to TCM when considering sub-fertility issues. The spleen, liver and kidney meridians each run into the feet, along with their partner meridians, the stomach, gall bladder and urinary bladder. It is worth noting, according to TCM, unless there is a mechanical or anatomical reason which prevents conception taking place then sub-fertility simply does not exist. Instead, there is considered an unbalanced system, with conception viewed as essentially a perfectly natural phenomenon accorded to a healthy human being.

Heightened emotional states are considered to *'eat up'* vitally required kidney energy according to TCM, and so the practice of meditation and focused energetic practices such as Qigong are widespread in the East; utilised to encourage calm in the mind and therefore the promotion of vital energy. Women experiencing sub-fertility issues can often report experiencing strong emotions of fear, anxiety, panic, frustration and even anger. According to TCM:

- **Fear** and **fright** are associated with **kidney** energy. The kidney is further associated with the reproductive hormones and ability to conceive. Any reduction in fear, according to TCM, can help to maintain vitality and strength in the vital kidney energy responsible for **conception**.

- **Anger** and **agitation** are associated with **liver** energy. The liver is further associated with the blood and **menstruation**.

- **Pensiveness** is associated with **spleen** energy. The spleen (and stomach) are further associated with extracting **nutrients** from the food we consume. In essence restoration of **personal energy**.

Women's Words

In order to better represent the multi-dimensional impact of the supportive reflexology package for this client group, in the following section I have opted to present a selection of phenomenological client statements taken from practice.

The DUB Sub-Fertility Client

Ruby, an otherwise healthy 34 year old woman, presented for reflexology after suffering several months of constant heavy menstrual bleeding. Dysfunctional uterine bleeding (DUB) is defined as abnormal uterine bleeding in the absence of organic disease. DUB usually presents as heavy menstrual bleeding (menorrhagia). A diagnosis of DUB can only be made once all other causes of abnormal or uterine bleeding have been excluded. The pathophysiology is largely unknown. Ruby had been recommended for ICSI (intra-cytoplasmic sperm injection), rather than IVF, because of an additional complication related to the presence of antibodies coating her husband's sperm.

Across the three months running up to the ICSI start date Ruby attended for reflexology on a weekly basis, receiving a full and firm treatment. Extra attention was given to the brain, pituitary, lungs, liver, adrenals and all of the reproductive reflex areas. Additionally, Ruby was asked to steep her feet in hot water daily, a practice often performed prior to reflexology in the East, in order to promote stimulation of the blood and to open the pores. Dietary considerations included generally promoting a more balanced healthy diet; focusing specifically on avoiding chemical additives and preservatives, so as to reduce impact on the liver. Ruby was also able to share her worries and frustrations within the confines of the therapeutic relationship, benefiting from encountering an empathic, supportive ear and appropriate education. Ruby's DUB markedly reduced within three weeks of sessions commencing, and her menstrual cycle began to settle into a more normal pattern, and she happily conceived naturally only a few weeks prior to her ICSI start date. We can now turn to Ruby's words to try and understand how she perceived her reflexology sessions may have helped her:

"Instead of obsessing about possible reasons for not conceiving, reflexology focused on the physical and mental issues that had put my body in turmoil, and supportive reflexology gave me a sense of perspective and hope. Stopping the contraceptive pill after 14 years left me with constant bleeding and hormonal irregularity, so that my body felt completely alien to me. Reflexology helped me to reclaim and understand my body, so that within weeks of starting treatment, I was healthier and happier than I had been in years. It took less than 10 weeks to prepare me to conceive naturally. Throughout the pregnancy, reflexology kept me grounded, focused and healthy. One of the most valuable

aspects of (the therapists) approach is her understanding that it is not possible to completely remove all potential barriers to conception. Giving up a stressful job was not an option for me, but the treatment helped me to understand how my body responded to that stress, and therefore gave me the power to choose a different response."

The IVF Client

Karen, an otherwise healthy 44 year old professional woman presented for treatment asking to be supported through her upcoming IVF protocol. Karen had already undergone seven full protocol IVF attempts (in addition to one frozen cycle and one IUI cycle) across a number of years. Now single and feeling as though her time and opportunities to be a parent were running out, Karen decided to opt for both donor eggs and sperm. Karen was to be supported though the initial stages of IVF by a respected UK unit, and her embryo transfer would take place abroad. It might be a fair to say Karen was understandably nervous and worried about the impending IVF. Her previous failures left her emotional drained and familiar with disappointment. Karen was anxious to do all she possibly could to ensure a successful outcome at what would probably be her final attempt at IVF. Karen attended for reflexology for 14 weeks prior to embryo transfer. Across this time she seemed to take particular encouragement from the rationale presented regarding the potential effects of the HPA axis on conception, and this information prompted Karen to start to make more time in her life centred upon better self care, relaxation and promoting calm. Sessions were utilised to draw encouragement and reassurance from the therapist and Karen seemed to adopt a more philosophical attitude as the weeks went moved on. We can now turn to Karen's words to try and understand more about what she was experiencing:

"I am a 44 year old GP who had been trying to conceive for 8 years. I am pleased that I rang a few months before treatment was due to begin and essentially we had our first consultation on the telephone. The therapist spent about 40 minutes asking questions, talking through my history and about her positive experiences of helping women to conceive. At the time of my first appointment (the therapist) spent a further hour and a

half with me talking and the performing the reflexology treatment. I felt very relaxed after the treatment, but it was different from other reflexology experiences. I felt more alert and found the therapist spent time finding out more about me, my experiences and giving me very positive messages and challenging some of my negative thoughts. I went for reflexology regularly from then on, usually about once a week, but sometimes less frequently. I was advised to increase my protein intake and that would help with energy levels. Over the weeks I was starting to look less tired and wrung out. The therapist talked about the negative effect of stress hormones on the uterus, and the reduction in the chances of embryos implanting, which made a lot of sense. Because of my treatments I realised how stressed and deflated I had become as a result of the repeated failures. The therapist gave me faith that the treatment could work if we got my body and mind in a confident state and ready to receive a pregnancy. I was going to be away in Cyprus for the treatment and (the therapist) was very reassuring that not having reflexology for a couple of weeks would not impact negatively on the outcome, because we had already helped my body and mind into the right place to conceive. With a previous practitioner I would have rushed back up from embryo transfer to have acupuncture, which seemed to add to the stress and the pressure of the whole process. I felt relaxed as I left for the transfer and managed to deal with the whole experience well. I had had so many negative tests previously that fear was stopping me taking the pregnancy test when the time came. I was too scared of the outcome. I arrived for reflexology and (the therapist) without quite saying it told me I was being ridiculous (something my friends had not quite managed to do) and that the outcome would be the same whether I checked or not, and it may well be positive. I did the test there and then and then sat having reflexology feeling stunned by the positive result and constantly checking the stick that I could not put down. The therapist offered that I did not have the treatment as she was sure I had plenty of people to phone, but I wanted to have it. A long journey! I am now 32 weeks pregnant with twins - a boy and a girl! Both are to doing well on the scans and are over 3 and a half pounds each. I am sure reflexology has played a significant part in preparing me for this pregnancy and ensuring that my body and mind were in the right place to receive a pregnancy. The therapists treatment, support, advice, stories of her life experiences and good humour have all played a vital role in helping me to finally become pregnant. Something that I thought would never happen. I am eternally grateful."

Clearly from a quantitative standpoint there are several different factors in this case which may have individually or collectively contributed to Karen's positive result - not limited to the use of donor eggs and sperm; embryo transfer taking place abroad, the inclusion of supportive reflexology, and even increased levels self care. It would be fairly impossible therefore to *quantify* the effect of each individual factor however Karen's positive *perception* of supportive reflexology seems to be clear and demonstrable within her words.

The ICSI Client

Cassie, an otherwise healthy 31 year professional woman, presented for treatment wishing to be supported through an upcoming third ICSI cycle. Cassie had been trying to conceive for over five years, previously treated pharmaceutically with both clomifene and metformin. Additionally, Cassie underwent an ovarian drilling procedure, as well as three unstimulated, and two stimulated IUI procedures. Cassie presented weekly for treatment for two months prior to the start of her third ICSI cycle and continued with weekly sessions throughout her ICSI treatment. In Cassie's words:

"I'd always been sceptical of complementary therapies, all the yin and yang, funny smells and gobbledegook terms, but this was something different. Never before had I met a person before who instilled such positivity. For the first time in a long time I felt like someone finally understood me, understood our situation and genuinely wanted to help. The therapist's down-to-earth and truthful approach was something we hadn't experienced during treatment so far. Everything else was very generic, and we were just a number in a very large group with a common theme; unexplained infertility. The therapists approach was different; she dug deep to learn more about me as a person and alongside the reflexology the work was heavily complemented by a genuine desire to learn about the feelings I was experiencing, and the desire to try to unravel the negative thoughts spinning round in my head. After my first session, I genuinely had a lot of

respect for her work: not only did she clearly know her subject areas, but she also respected the views I held, and the concerns that had developed over my medical treatment. Throughout the coming weeks I learnt to open up about things I'd never really shared before, and own up to the feelings I had; laying them on the table and mentally smashing the negative ones with a huge hammer. Rather than concentrating on the thoughts placed in our minds by our medical professionals, I began to realise that all the inconclusive testing was actually a positive thing. My mindset changed and it was no longer about consultants not being able to find a real cause for our constant failures, it became more about the fact that they couldn't find a cause because there just wasn't anything wrong; there was no reason for the treatments not to work. This became my new outlook. The NHS waiting times between treatments were long but I used this time to let the therapist work her magic and get me into the most positive and relaxed mindset possible. Don't get me wrong, there were still moments I sat quietly on a night and asked myself if I was living in the real world, or was I letting myself be led into a place where fairies danced and where everything was going to be nice and perfect. Physically, my menstrual cycles started to change and became less of a hassle. My partner was finally able to take his tin-hat off and felt safe I wasn't going to throw things at his head every month. As our final IVF cycle loomed, I actually felt more in control than I had throughout any other treatment. My partner and I made all the decisions around our treatment; not the nurses, nor the consultants. I was in a positive place and didn't experience the pressure I'd felt on myself during other cycles. January 2013 was a new start and our treatment went relatively smoothly, just as the previous cycles had. The outcome though was unexpected. After over 60 months of unbearable disappointment, seeing a single blue line each and every time, we finally saw 2 very definite blue lines. Now, at 18 weeks, with 2 strong beating hearts and a beautiful rounded bump we feel utterly blessed. The pain and heartache of the last few years is still fresh in our minds, but the feeling of joy as the flutters begin makes everything so worth it. We are incredibly lucky, and don't take anything for granted at the moment but this amazing feeling of waking up each morning knowing our lives are changing in such a wonderful way is a feeling that cannot be put into words. As for the yin and the yang, the funny smells and the gobbledegook; which actually makes perfect sense, we're now firm believers. To be understood as person, rather than counted as an unwanted statistic makes every difference".

The Unexplained Sub-Fertility Client

Esther, an otherwise healthy 36 year old woman, presented for treatment hoping to be supported in her desire to become pregnant for the third time after recently having experienced miscarriage. Esther was anxious to add to her family, particularly wishing to conceive a sibling for her young son, and it would be fair to say feelings of panic had set in. Over the coming weeks Esther made changes to her diet (ensuring to eat regularly to promote balanced bloods sugar levels, and ensure restorative energy supply) whilst the reflexology sessions were focused towards drawing encouragement and support from the therapist. In Esther's words:

"After nearly three years of trying to conceive my cycle was a bit of a mess and my emotions were all over the place. I had managed to conceive a few times, but each had led to an early loss. My head was in a knot of thoughts that would go round and round, so loud and noisy it was hard to sleep or think straight and everything seemed to come back to one thought; will I have another baby? I started reflexology desperate for some relief from the symptoms of clomifene and hopefully to increase the chances of getting pregnant. I think more than anything I hoped that the reflexology might just help me feel a little more peaceful. I had reflexology once a week and we talked through my feelings, and how I was dealing with things. I found the hour long sessions provided intense relaxation, and it would lead to a better night's sleep. At home I followed the advice to improve my diet, but the best thing I was advised to do was to be kind to myself. I focused on what would make me feel better and what I enjoyed. After the first month of treatment the flow of my period was much improved, and didn't feel so congested. The PMT symptoms were reduced and instead of taking multiple high strength pain killers, I only needed two tablets across my whole period; which hadn't happened since I was 13. I attended for reflexology for four months and during that time my moods continued to improve - my husband, a non believer in complementary therapies even commented that I was 'better to do with'. I felt a freedom in my mind that allowed me to see things more

clearly. I began to believe in my body; that it could and would get pregnant. I even spent my saved up IVF money on a new car! I got a new job to help reduce stress, but before I could even start the new job two lines appeared on a pregnancy test! Reflexology helped me stay calm and relax during the anxious first few weeks, and at eight weeks pregnant I had my first scan and saw two little hearts beating away. Now at 28 weeks both are growing well and weigh 2lb 9 each, we are really looking forward to their arrival."

The Endometriosis Client

Jane a 35 year old woman presented after a friend recommended reflexology. Jane had been diagnosed with stage four endometriosis, and after three largely unsuccessful laparoscopies was still in severe pain, suffering exhaustion and struggling to return to work after a year off sick. Jane had been informed by her consultant that natural conception was unlikely, although the thought of embarking on IVF treatment was still far in the future for Jane. Her immediate concern was pain. A plan was constructed which included making dietary changes in an attempt to promote less strain on liver function (*blood and menstrual problems link directly to liver function, according to the principles of TCM*), as well as introducing more protein and fluids. At the first session the pathology of Jane's feet was acutely sensitive, and the pressure therapy deeply uncomfortable in some areas despite very gentle finger and thumb movements. Over the weeks this acute sensitivity lessened, directly in line with an improvement in Jane's general levels of pain, and an associated reduction in the use of topical analgesia (thus promoting a less stressed liver). Jane's words:

"After an intensive course of reflexology I found I was better able to deal with my pain levels and felt emotionally stronger. I returned to work four days a week, fairly quickly. Within three months of starting the treatments I was delighted to find I was pregnant. I would recommend reflexology to anyone experiencing similar problems. I am convinced I would never have felt better, nor fallen pregnant without (it)."

As is fairly common in some women with endometriosis, pregnancy and a period of breast feeding resulted in a vast reduction of Jane's returning symptoms post pregnancy. Jane continues to uphold her dietary considerations and promote good circulation in an attempt to reduce the symptoms returning.

The Repeated Miscarriage Client

Paula, an otherwise healthy 31 year old woman presented for treatment after two miscarriages across a two years period. Paula heard about reflexology from a friend and thought it might help. Despite an obvious improvement in Paula's fertility across the treatment period (Paula became pregnant and miscarried a further three times in 12 months), Paula and her husband, crushed by yet another disappointment, eventually concluded their journey to conceive naturally had come to an end. Paula and her husband have subsequently gone on to adopt two beautiful children and as a family today they could not be happier. In Paula's words:

"It is hard to sum up in a few words how much reflexology helped me when I was going through my journey to becoming a parent, but here goes! Physically I felt after each consultation that I was completely relaxed (driving home was always a bit of an effort!). Throughout the duration of the treatment I did become pregnant several times but sadly these pregnancies were not meant to be. Emotionally, when I first met (the therapist) it was like speaking to an old friend but someone who really understood what we were going through and truly empathised. I had confidence (in the treatment) but never assumed that the outcome would be a baby, even though that's was what we hoped for. In the end we have two beautiful boys, through adoption. I believe that in attending for reflexology treatment regularly (the therapist) kept my mind in good health, which kept me in a position to adopt. Trying to have a family is all consuming and it can be hard to see anything outside that when you are stuck in the middle of it – reflexology managed to achieve that. I will always be eternally grateful for all the help and support on our journey even though we are not good for baby statistics!!! I am so pleased our journey has been what it is. I have never been so happy and proud to be a mum of our two gorgeous, loving sons – this was our path and (reflexology) helped us on our way."

Despite her painful and traumatic difficulties Paula's experiences remain a valid example of how supportive reflexology can benefit sub-fertility clients. Paula's increased levels of fertility across the session duration, despite the further sad loss of these pregnancies (*possibly owning to genetic factors given a similar gestation period at which each of the pregnancies was lost*) perhaps demonstrates reflexology can support women to conceive naturally. Paula's experiences also perhaps demonstrate the important and valuable supportive and emotional benefits to be gained from engaging with a confident and empathic reflexology practitioner. Therapeutic support stemming from the application of reflexology is perhaps well demonstrated in this case as extending far beyond the pressure therapy alone.

Undoubtedly, my role s a therapist within this example involved heavy ethical responsibility. Although confident to re-engage with Paula, post an appropriate recovery period, reflexology was resumed after careful discussion with the client. It was Paula who led the way, owning her own experience, and my role was entirely supportive.

Summary

When reflecting on the words of the women the overall *existential* value derived from receiving supportive relational reflexology seems to have been experienced as wholly beneficial to the health and well-being of this particular client group. **Support**, **advice** and **education** seem to be some of the most highlighted benefits identified, as well as feelings of being **understood**. Better quality of **sleep** and **relaxation** are also mentioned, as well as more **positive feelings**. Practiced to a high professional standard, ethically, and mindful of the delicate interacting processes connecting mind and body, supportive reflexology seems to have proved immensely beneficial to each of these women. The women's words also highlight some of the deep emotional frustrations experienced by the sub-fertility group, and how emotional vulnerability is fairly common place. High levels of practitioner competence, in addition to sufficient levels of self development are therefore of paramount importance when engaging therapeutically with this group. This is probably this most important, all encompassing event to take place in a woman's life. As reflexology practitioners we must remain mindful of that that all important fact, and ensure at all times our clients remain safe and are cared for with the utmost respect.

Sub-fertility is not a field of holistic dreams, nor is it a field filled with magic or false promises. Supportive reflexology is a professional and ethically driven field, requiring only excellence, honestly, and genuineness. Human interactions, touch, support and knowledge are the collective elements responsible for any '*magic*' taking place. The clients make the changes that really matter, and the professional practitioner's role is to demonstrate through the medium of reflexology, and the supportive therapeutic relationship, how those changes might be made. Working with the whole person provides the practitioner with an opportunity to offer:

- A supportive therapeutic space in which client can share their worries and concerns, should they wish to.
- Reflexology stimulation and the benefit of interpersonal touch.
- Appropriate education promoting the concept of client autonomy and self-directed change.

Supportive reflexology, when administered by well educated and ethically driven practitioners, may well offer many sub-fertility clients the perfect complementary therapeutic modality in which both body and mind-set might be encouraged towards achieving more regular instances of the relaxation state - therefore promoting provision of the *hospitable womb*.

That is mind, body, spirit.

TCM Philosophy and Reflexology

"Massaging the foot in spring strengthens immunity; in summer relieves heat; in autumn prevents constipation and in winter warms the body."

- Hao Tuo Cheats

Eastern attitudes relating to health and the nature of the universe have remained relatively unaltered across many thousands of years. The absence of influence stemming from classical Greek thinking within Eastern culture means concepts have remained more faithful to their ancient, mystical origins. Initially dismissed on mass by Western thinkers as simply philosophical and ethnological traditions, unfortunately assumption alone suggested these traditions were fundamentally scientifically flawed and defective. Eastern philosophies are however universally clear in stating both time and space are inseparably connected, with each other, and with other aspects of the universe, such as the concepts of movement and energy. Eastern philosophies are also presently being considered by many modern physicists as corresponding more closely to modern scientific thinking than was ever imagined possible.

Traditional Chinese medicine dates back to around 2900 BC and was said to be founded by the part mythical creature Fu Hsi - first responsible for describing the concept of Qi, and the universal principles of yin and yang. Indications stemming from writings such as the Huang Ti Nei Ching (The Yellow Emperor's Treatise on Internal Medicine, c. 770-467BC) demonstrate clearly early Chinese cultures believed man to be a perfect image of the cosmos and absolutely attuned to nature.

"Man instinctively and collectively understood and lived in accordance with its fundamental forces" (Graham, 1990)

At the heart of TCM is the tenet that the root cause of illness, not just the symptoms must be treated; a truly holistic approach, acknowledging every aspect of the person (their body, mind and spirit) as part of one complete interacting circle, rather than loosely connected pieces to be treated individually.

Reflexology and TCM Philosophy

The first writings referencing foot diagnosis in Chinese culture can be found in the Huang Ti Nei Ching. However foot massage remained a relatively minor branch of TCM until the time of the Ming and Qing Dynasties, when the physician Hau Tuo (145-208AD) coined the form 'Zu Xin Theory'.

"Because of the simplicity and practicality (hand and foot massage) has long been very wide spread among the ordinary people of China, although it was not admitted to the honoured ranks of classical tradition of medicine due to certain historical reasons." (Genwei & DongFang, 2006)

During the Ming and Qing Dynasties TCM massage was developed and combined with the theory of meridians and acupoints. Points on the hands and feet were frequently used within TCM massage to treat disease. In China today reflexology is still practiced from within the holistic principles of TCM, and combines with the clinical experience of modern medicine.

A TCM Perspective on Health and Wellbeing

According to the ancient Chinese there are meridians (or energy pathways) running through the body – linked to various organs and functions. When Qi in the body is able to run through the meridians smoothly and unhindered, good health prevails. When Qi becomes blocked or obstructed however, illness can occur therefore treatment according to TCM is principally concerned with normalising energy flow in the body.

- There are 23 acupoints on the **hand** – 9 on the palm and 14 on the top of the hand associated with the lung, large intestine, heart and small intestine meridians.

- There are 33 acupoints located on the **feet** associated with the spleen, stomach, liver, gall bladder, kidney and bladder meridians.

Within TCM the feet are viewed as a fundamental source of treatment and regarded as the roots of the body. The foot acupressure points are believed to reflect various disease states in the body. It is believed disease states can be alleviated by stimulation because of an intimate relationship between:

- The feet
- The viscera (internal organs)
- The meridians (energy pathways)
- The blood
- The Three Treasures in TCM – Life Sustaining Energies

JING - nutritive essence, essence, refined, perfected, extract, spirit, demon, sperm, seed

The Chinese word for essence, specifically referring to kidney essence. The Jing is said to be the material basis for the physical body. The Jing nourishes fuels and cools the body and is the carrier of our genetic heritage. The production of semen in males, and menstrual blood (and pregnancy) in females can place strains on the levels of Jing in the body. Given individuals are said to be genetically gifted with a finite amount of Jing, therefore efficient replenishing of energy in the body is of paramount importance in order to maintain good health. According to TCM the restorative energy required for maintaining good health is sourced from food Qi, and prolonged by breath Qi (exercise and meditation).

The Chinese therefore believe healthy Jing is not only important regarding conception, for example, but also in maintaining general good health and longevity in the individual.

QI - vitality, energy, force, air, vapor, breath, spirit, vigor

Qi can be translated as vital energy that when free flowing and unrestricted, reflects in a healthy body. Qi flows through pathways called meridians and is most associated with the liver and and spleen systems. Qi animates our bodies, allowing for the movement of breath in and out of our lungs, and the movement of blood through the vessels. In TCM blood is considered as a fluid not only confined to blood vessels, but also believed to run through the meridians of the body.

SHEN - spirit, soul, mind, god, deity, supernatural being

Shen resides in the heart and mind. A healthy, vibrant person is described as having good Shen; often considered to be reflected through shining, twinkling eyes, and viewed as an emanation of spiritual radiance, and an enlightened and forgiving heart and mind. Metaphorically, if we imagine Jing as the wax and wick of a candle and Qi its flame, then Shen might be seen as the radiance given off by the flame. In the same way as light from the candle is dependent on wax, wick and flame, so healthy Shen is dependent on the cultivation of good Jing and Qi. A balanced and healthy body and mind therefore enables the radiant spirit to shine.

Understanding Qi

According to TCM Qi is the fundamental energy of nature and the universe. Each movement or change in the physical world can be related to movement and changes of Qi. Similarly, everything that happens inside the body is driven by the flow of Qi. TCM theory states in order to maintain good health the body must have enough Qi, and that the Qi must be free to flow throughout the body unhindered, thus ensuring all the vital organs and tissues are supplied with the energy required to function correctly.

If levels of Qi in the body drop due to poor nutrition or heightened emotional states, or if the flow of Qi becomes blocked or hindered, the body is considered likely to experience dis-ease and poor health might be expected in the systems and their functions.

Jing (source Qi) - This Jing is inherited genetically at conception. Source Qi resides in the kidney and from there flows throughout the body via the meridian system. Source Qi provides the vital organs with the energy to function properly and efficiently. Source Qi requires nourishment which is obtained from essential Qi.

Essential Qi - This nourishing Qi forms when Qi from the lungs and Qi from food essence combine. The essential or pectoral Qi is stored in the chest and has two principle purposes: to support the heart (circulation) and lungs (respiration).

Defensive Qi - This Qi is formed from food essence and provides immune support for the body. It resides in the muscles, skin and hair. Defensive Qi holds the ability to regulate the skin for example, helping to control the temperature of body tissue.

Nutrient Qi - This Qi again originates from food essence. Nutrient Qi resides and circulates in the blood vessels, and is responsible for generating new blood and for nourishing existing blood, as it is circulated by the body.

Zang Fu Theory

According to the tradition of TCM the theory of Zang-Fu defines the composition of internal organs as well as the energy systems that link each organ to one another, and in turn to the whole of the body. The theory describes the production, transformation, and maintenance of the four basic life materials (essence, Qi, blood and body fluids) by the Zang-Fu organs. The study of the organ system includes both the physiology of the specific organs, as well as their related tissues. States of dis-ease might be explained as conditions of excessive, deficient, or stagnant energy (Qi) within the organ system. The yang organs function to transform and store Qi are associated with the interior of the body. The fu organs function to clear the body of waste and associated with the exterior of the body.

Seven Emotions in TCM

One fundamental difference existing between TCM and the Western medical view of health might be the inclusion of, and importance placed upon, an individual's emotional state. TCM considers emotions as intertwined within the principles of good health and medicine. The Zang-Fu associations demonstrate certain organs are related to emotional activities; the heart is related to joy, the liver to anger, the spleen to pensiveness, the lungs to anxiety, and the kidneys to fear. According to TCM, excessive, prolonged emotional states are considered a major internal cause of disease. Emotional activity is generally considered as a normal physiological response to stimuli from the external environment. Under normal conditions, emotions are not considered to induce illness or weakness in the body. However, when emotions become elevated or prolonged in their duration, the individual can become prone to injury of the internal organs and therefore more susceptible to disease.

Whilst Western medicine tends to stress the more psychological aspects of psychosomatic ailments, the pathological consequence of emotional states impacting internal organs is of primary concern to the TCM practitioner.

The seven emotions according to TCM are:

- **Joy** - In TCM, joy refers to a state of agitation or overexcitement, rather than passive happiness. Over-stimulation of joy can lead to problems associated with the heart and is connected with feelings of agitation, insomnia and palpitations.

- **Anger** - Anger according to TCM encapsulates a whole range of emotions including resentment, irritability, and frustration, and it is believed an excess of rich (toxic) blood can encourage anger in the individual. Anger is believed to affect the liver primarily resulting in a stagnation of liver Qi, leading to liver energy rising to the head, often resulting in headaches, dizziness and even high blood pressure. The liver meridian is also believed to run directly through the uterine cavity and is believed to be responsible for providing a woman's menstrual bleed each month.

- **Anxiety** - Anxiety is believed to cause injury to the lungs according to TCM and so shallow and irregular breathing are considered a symptom of anxiety. Anxiety also causes problems in the fu organ associated with the lung, the large intestine. For example, over-anxious people are prone to ulcerative colitis and IBS.

- **Pensiveness** - According to TCM, pensiveness is considered to result from thinking too much, or excessive mental stimulation and the organ most at risk is the spleen. A deficiency of spleen Qi can also result in feelings of worry fatigue, lethargy, and an inability to concentrate.

- **Grief** - Grief, according to TCM is also associated with the lungs. Unresolved chronic grief can create disharmony which in turn is believed to interfere with the lungs function of circulating Qi around the body.

- **Fear** - Again fear is considered as a perfectly normal human emotion, however when fear becomes chronic and the perceived cause cannot be directly addressed, then disharmony is believed to occur in the kidneys. In cases of extreme fright, the kidney's ability to hold Qi may be impaired leading to involuntary urination (think Interstitial Cystitis).

- **Fright** - Fright is distinguished from fear according to TCM by its sudden, unexpected nature. Fright is considered to initially affect the heart, but if it persists it can become a more conscious fear and move to the kidney.

The information presented in this blog has been collated so as to provide the professional reflexology practitioner with an additional health philosophy to consider in practice.TCM philosophy, and in particular the principles of Zang Fu, can often provide us with potential links between physiological disorders and possible associated emotional states. The information can be used to better inform the practitioner, and can also be used reflectively, where appropriate, with clients.

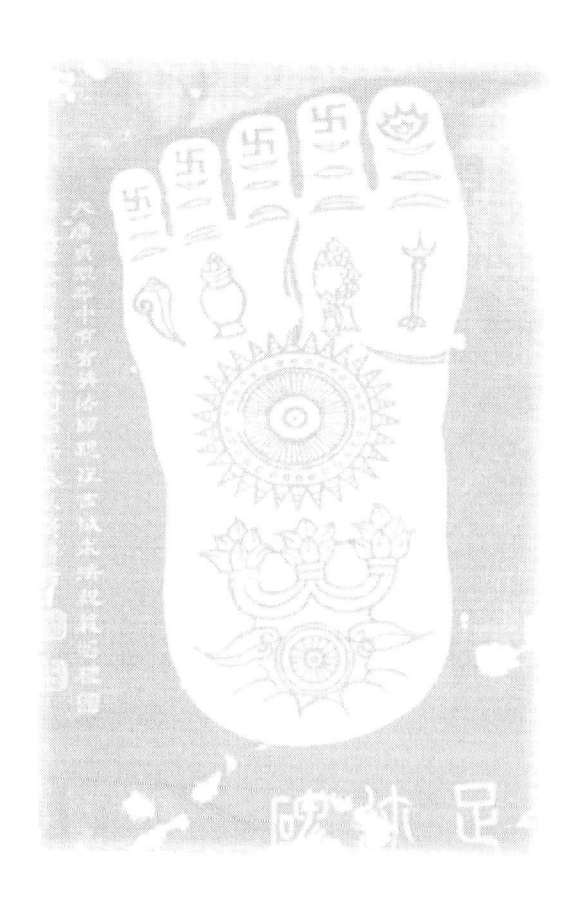

Zang Fu Table:

Zang Organ	Associated Fu Organ	Sensory Organ	Associated Emotion	Associated Systems and Functions
Spleen	Stomach	Mouth	Pensiveness	Spleen energy is responsible for extracting nutrients from the food we consume and converting those nutrients into blood and Qi. Meridian active between 7-9am & 9-11am. Linked to the stomach and upper part of the digestion. Mouth ulcers, sickness (reversed Spleen/stomach Qi is often associated with excessive emotions and a feeling of having something stuck in the throat impeding any feeling of being hungry.
Liver	Gall Bladder	Eyes	Anger and agitation	Associated with the blood and free flow of blood and qi around the body (circulation), liver function and toxin removal (the liver might be likened to a chemical processing factory), Meridians active between 11pm-1am & 1-3am. Associated with muscles (containing *blood*), the eyes, menstruation (liver 'gives' *blood* to the uterus each month). Links to headaches and migraines. Fibromyalgia, Poor circulation and the tendons.
Kidney	Urinary Bladder	Ears, genitals and anus	Fear and fright	Houses the 'Jing' (or life force energy) required for life and conception. Regulates the kidneys and urinary system. Meridians active between 3-5pm & 5-7pm. Associated with fright, fear and exhaustion. Links to the ears and so associated with vertigo, tinnitus and labyrinthitis. Regulates the elimination of toxins, the bones, hair, and reproductive hormones.
Lung	Large Intestine	Nose/Skin	Anxiety and grief	Linked to asthma, chest infections, IBS, eczema, rashes and flaky dry skin. Meridians active between 3-5am and 5-7am. The lung energy supports the heart and circulation and can be easily depleted as a result of stress or over-thinking. When lung energy is disturbed because clients are stressed they may have the tendency to wake around 4am (when the meridian is most active).
Heart	Small Intestine	Tongue	Joy	Linked to the vessels and vascular problems palpitations, chest discomfort, insomnia. sadness, anxiety issues, shyness, vascular Meridian active between 11am-1pm & 1-3pm

Relational Reflexology

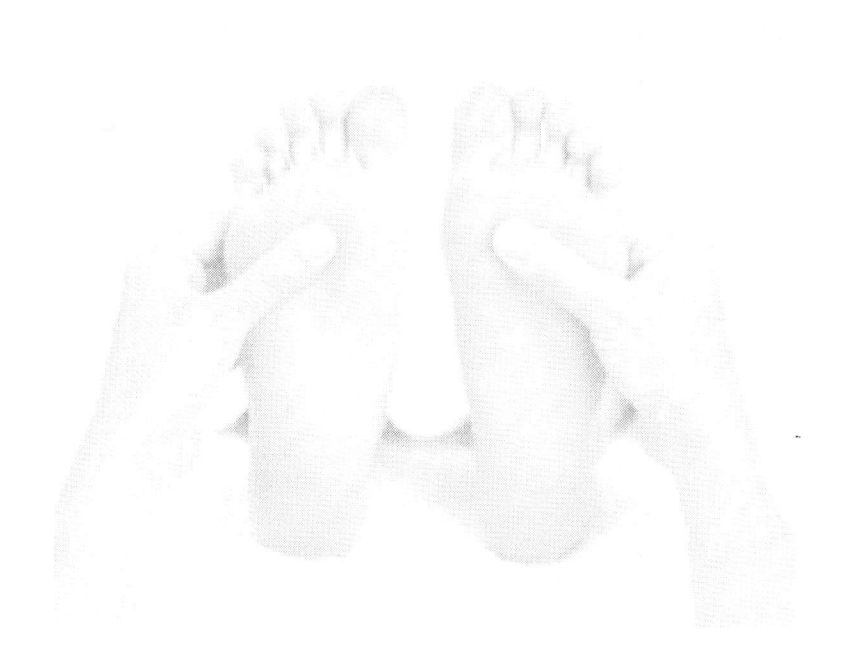

An Open Letter to the Beauty and Spa World

Dear Beauty and Spa World,

Prior to writing this letter I spent some time browsing through past threads in beauty therapy forums and social media groups. One theme I was able to identify within those threads centered round a sense of frustration regarding those individuals setting up beauty businesses when holding less than robust qualifications. Many of the comments in the forums seem to reveal a sense of unjustness and unfairness amongst beauty therapists as they find they begin to compare their own, often more expensive, in-depth training against that of the local competitor, qualified via some super cheap, fast track, minimalistic course.

Perhaps then it might be understandable to find professional reflexologists can often feel a similar sense of unfairness on finding their valuable complementary modality teachings dumbed down. Undoubtedly, within every industry there exist unethical, profit driven individuals, those for whom the bank balance seems to take precedence, or maybe it is the ego, or maybe both! Regardless, these often cheap, low contact, short courses certainly seem to be very present within the beauty industry, and so too are they still unfortunately present within reflexology.

As a growing CAM industry reflexology has taken some great leaps forward regarding professional standards. The minimum level of training for example, recognised by the established professional reflexology associations in the UK now stands at Level 3, with entry level training in some cases up to level 5.

Reflexology practitioner courses accredited by ABC, CIBTAC, City & Guilds, ITEC and VTCT, meet the standards required by the professional reflexology associations, and indeed the Complementary & Natural Health Council

(CNHC), set up with government funding in 2008, to act as the UK voluntary regulator for complementary healthcare practitioners.

"CNHC is accredited by the Professional Standards Authority for Health and Social Care as the holder of an Accredited Voluntary Register (AVR). CNHC is listed on PSA's directory of AVRs. Accreditation means that CNHC as an organisation has met the PSA's rigorous standards." (www.cnhc.org.uk)

In order to be eligible to be admitted to the CNHC Register, a complementary therapist must:

- Have undertaken a programme of education and training which meets, as a minimum, the National Occupational Standards and the core curriculum for the complementary therapy/discipline concerned where a core curriculum has been agreed.

or,

- Have achieved competency to the level of the National Occupational Standards for the complementary therapy/discipline concerned by means of relevant experience of at least three years and relevant training and been assessed as having met those standards.

Unfortunately, there are some individuals (here in the UK) who have opted to entirely ignore professional industry recommendations, and indeed the very existence of the reflexology core curriculum. Instead these individuals continue to offer to potential reflexology trainees the option of short, weekend, or distance learning courses – whilst readily assuring the uninitiated the course is of 'practitioner level'. There are also 'official bodies', some beauty industry based, and some entirely independent and self-governing (often correspondence type organisations) providing courses with 'accreditation' approval, in addition to some insurance companies providing cover. We continue to hear reports of fledgling reflexologists wasting valuable time and money on short courses, only latterly to find in order to proceed professionally, or to gain professional membership, they are required almost to start their reflexology training from scratch. In other cases some practitioners report they feel unprepared and inept to deal with the reality of a professional reflexology practice. These courses often also unfortunately continue to perpetuate the spreading of philosophical misinformation regarding reflexology – information not representative of the opinion of our wider professional educational community. How can this type of short reflexology training ever be deemed worthy of any form of accreditation when it seems to fall so very short of meeting the recommended industry standards? Our professional reflexology associations are continually attempting to inform potential CAM focused trainees on how best to source good quality reflexology training, which brings me to purpose of this open letter to the members of the beauty and spa world:

That is to respectfully make three requests of therapists who choose to engage in cross-over beauty/holistic work.

1. That those therapists who wish to incorporate reflexology into their professional repertoire complete a recognised Level 3 reflexology qualification. RReflexology is a wonderful healing modality, and frankly, the more well qualified reflexologists around – the better! If you can, try to find an experienced tutor. One who can really teach you the true art of reflexology, one who can, through experience, teach you more than just the location of a particular reflex. Try to locate a tutor who will encourage you to work therapeutically with the whole person.

2. That those therapists who have no real desire to further their reflexology training, but do wish to incorporate hand, or foot massage into their beauty work, consider supporting the reflexology industry by making a clear intellectual and advertising distinction between foot massage and professional reflexology.

3. Finally, please help to support the reflexology industry by boycotting all short, weekend or distance learning reflexology practitioner level training programmes.

Reflexology is a wonderfully complex, multi-dimensional complementary modality and the impact of the reflexology package can be powerful and often transformative for clients. Our practitioners are increasingly engaging in good quality research, and we are beginning to fully grasp the multi-layered complexities of the reflexology package. A good reflexologist works with people, not just feet. Reflexology is about touch, pressure, appropriate knowledge, spoken and unspoken communications, philosophy, intuition, intimate human interaction, support, care, and sometimes even guidance. Reflexology is so very much more than a relaxing foot massage.

If you are a cross-over beauty/spa type therapist perhaps you might consider sharing this open letter with your colleagues? Please help to support our CAM industry protect the reputation of reflexology, by following and recommending the educational standards currently set out by the professional reflexology industry.

Respectfully,

A Professional Reflexologist

Hope and Closing Reflections

"Everything that is done in this world is done by hope."

- Martin Luther

There are times I have cried with my clients, and there are times I have laughed. I have offered encouragement and support, and where possible, helped to illuminate future paths. I have listened, empathised, touched, and advised. As a professional reflexologist I doubt I am alone in that. What defines *therapy*? In many ways the word seems to have become heavily aligned with mental health issues and psychologically based interventions. In fact, the word therapy originally stems from the Greek word *'therapeia'* meaning *'healing'*. I personally firmly believe any form of therapy (or healing) should be a journey of exploration and learning, otherwise I'm not entirely sure it should be contextualised as *therapy*. I believe without client engagement in the process there is only passiveness and a procedure, and certainly, with stressed and anxious clients, that stance represents the difference between an hour's reflexology and all its many benefits, and experiencing that, in addition to gaining personal insight and strategies for use outside of that hour.

My own journey as a therapist has been a joy and a revelation. I recall my first tentative steps and my feelings of achievement as I began to master my routine and technique, and started to feel more confident the reflexology map was firmly imprinted in my mind. As I relaxed and began to step back from some of my initial anxieties (mostly centred around getting it right), I found I was better able to appreciate some of the complex transformations occurring within the walls of my therapy room and I began to make my own mental notes.

Possibly because of my auricular acupuncture training, I began to categorise clients according to condition type fairly quickly; *blood related conditions, anxiety related conditions, chronic internalised conditions*, etc. Soon I became aware of subtle correlations within personality types related to each group - *the sad client, the childlike client, the toxic agitated client*, and *the anxious client*. Before long I added a new category to my internal indexing system, *the cascade client*! You might know this client type? As the initial presenting issue seems to shift, another quickly appears in its place, and then another? Around this time I also began to accept that some of my reflexology clients seemed more focused upon engaging pro-actively in their health than others. Over time, this realisation helped me to understand that no matter how powerful reflexology might be, or how positive my intention, the end result mostly lay in close alignment with the level of client engagement in the overall healing process.

I started to utilise mindfulness principles and the Pooh psychology concepts in my work, teaching abdominal breathing exercises and offering light hearted character interpretations to my clients. Pooh psychology is a concept I have be aware of for many years, stretching back to my years as a children's nanny. Just about everyone understands Pooh and his friends; from eight years to eighty years! Just about everyone giggles when you offer the story, and most people learn something. Mindfulness is a lovely philosophy, and very easily learned. Try everyday to be *present* in your own life! Try not to get lost in thoughts and images of yesterday, tomorrow, or next week. Try instead to sense, feel and experience within each moment. As we begin to simplify our thoughts, so to we often begin to simplify our lives. This means we also tend to become more focused on engaging in activities that really make us smile inside. It's all helpful.

There really is no fixed requirement for *therapy* to be serious or deep, in fact too much serious and deep is often what brought the client to reflexology in the first place. Therapy does though require structure, philosophical and educational context, and client participation. Perhaps most crucially therapy requires solid professional boundaries. Personally, I have every faith in the abilities of those particular human beings choosing to spend their time and money training in complementary therapies such as reflexology, but I also strongly believe we can always *choose* to develop our professional skills further. I hope therefore some of the information in this book might prompt readers to turn their attention to enhancing the important relational side of their reflexology practice.

I've been asked a few times to describe the manner in which I work the feet. I'm afraid my reply may not appear terribly interesting, principally because my method is rather simple. I work *whatever* I find with *any* particular person, on *any* particular day, using a fairly firm pressure. I have remained pretty faithful to the routine I was originally taught (*thank you Kathleen*), mostly because it allows me to cover every part of the foot in a fairly systematic fashion. I tend to work the feet twice, returning to rework any area I feel may require a little more attention. I try not to think about reflexology too technically if I am entirely honest. I prefer to *feel* my way around.

The articles in the book clearly represent my own unique perspective on the reflexology package. The book represents my offering to the collective reflexology table - an offering to be shared, considered, digested and possibly even spat out by some! Of course, there are some practitioners who will remain uninterested in developing the relational aspects of their practice. They will probably tell you reflexology should be a meditation, or that it should *always* be performed in silence. Often too they will tell you that *their* clients simply don't want to talk.

"Psychological or interpersonal processes inevitably form part of all treatment encounters." (Mitchell and Cormack, 1998)

Actually, what is more likely to be occurring is some of these clients will be aware of unspoken, implicit messages within the body language of the practitioner that say, *"I'm sorry, but I'm really not very comfortable talking with you."* Of course not every client wishes to talk, and it should *always* be the client who chooses how to use the reflexology space. However, when an emotionally vulnerable client walks into a therapy room with either stand alone emotional content, or content accompanying a physiological issue, and decides *not* to share their story, rest assured, it is fairly likely they simply do not trust the practitioner in front of them wants to hear.

"If you work with the body using touch, your hands will have learned how to listen to the tissues, or to energy flow. What would it be like to listen to the words a person says with the same sensitivity and single channel attention?"(Fox, 2008)

Perhaps my greatest hope is that the information presented might help to build confidence in practice, to join unconnected dots, to provide layering and context, and offer new insight. I hope too some of the impact might be to draw attention to the important concept of *brain health*, and also to the concept that sometimes as we journey through life we may find we're requiring of a little support, a little strength, a push in the right direction, and that now might be the time to acknowledge professional reflexologists are stepping into *that* particular role quite successfully every day.

My intention has always been to highlight the role of the therapeutic relationship in reflexology, and to try and widen the general viewpoint. Central to the depth and success of any therapeutic relationship is the practitioner. Much has been written about the power of reflexology, very little is mentioned about the power of the *reflexologist*. I hope in some small way some of the articles in this book might begin to alter that reality and help to highlight and champion the important role of the professional reflexologist. I am certainly aware of a collective engaging on a constant learning curve, oozing dedication, and displaying a genuine desire to help and support their clients.

I believe reflexology, in the hands of well informed and dedicated practitioners, may well emerge as one of the most positively impacting complementary therapies available, and I use the word *therapy* consciously, in its fullest possible sense, to represent not only the physical component of the modality, but also to loudly acknowledge the vastly integral role of the practitioner within the reflexology package. The professional reflexologist is a quietly dedicated individual. As a collective, their depth of caring, positive intention in touch, support, dedication, knowledge, and empathy are helping to positively transform the lives of reflexology clients every single day. The value contained within that important work is perhaps immeasurable.

It would seem many of our collective reflexology interventions may be impacting many of the much older mammalian parts of the brain. The areas linked to intuition, emotion, learning, memory, survival, and homeostasis. As the more cognitively focused, task performing area of our brains evolved; the thinking, forward projecting parts, perhaps human beings simply stopped day dreaming quite so much? Perhaps in our modern world there is entirely too much *doing* and simply not enough *being*? Science informs us our brain utilises the relaxed, default, day-dreaming place to recover, repair, gather strength, and to deal with much of our uncategorised emotional content. It seems this is a valuable place we should be permitting our brains to visit more often?

Evolution may have presented us with a means of *fast track accessing* the default network of the brain (and therefore the body) via the feet. That, coupled with the support of a well educated, self aware, confident therapist can be a transformative combination. Reflexology is perhaps the *only* complementary therapy so constructed to meet the many complex multi-dimensional requirements of those individuals focused upon improving their health and well-being.

Perhaps also, we can be reliably assured, the innate intuition residing within human beings, wired by evolution to recognise the healing worth of touch, relaxation, reboot and repair, will *always* find therapeutic value in reflexology.

Relational Reflexology

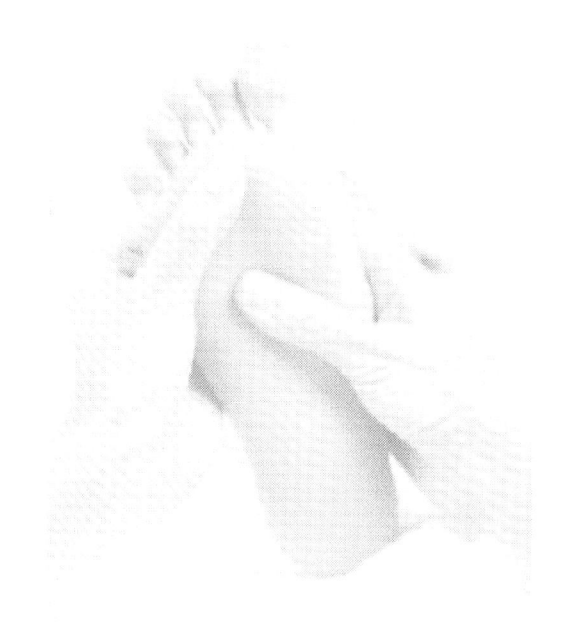

References

Bagheri-Nesami, M., Shorofi, S., Zargar, N., Sohrabi, M., Gholipour-Baradari, A., & Khalilian, A. (2014). The effects of foot reflexology massage on anxiety in patients following coronary artery bypass graft surgery: a randomised controlled trial. Complement Ther Clin Pract. 2014 Feb; 20(1):42-7.

Balk, J., Catov, J., Horn, B., Gecsi, K., & Wakim, A. (2009). The relationship between perceived stress, acupuncture, and pregnancy rates among IVF patients: A pilot study. Elsevier.

Beddoe, A. E., & Lee, K. A. (2008). Mind-body interventions during pregnancy. Journal of Obstetric, Gynaecological and Neonatal Nursing.

Beddoe, A. E., Paul Yang, C. P., Kennedy, H. P., Weiss, S. J., & Lee, K. A. (2009). The effects of mindfulness-based yoga during pregnancy on maternal psychological and physical distress. Journal of Obstetric, Gynaecological and Neonatal Nursing.

Biola, J,M., Hernando, H., & Esteban B. (2011). Environmental Triggers and Epigenetic Deregulation in Autoimmune Disease. Discov Med 12(67):535-545.

Birk, T. J. (2000). The Effects of massage Therapy Alone and in Combination with Other Complementary Therapies on Immune System Measures and Quality of Life in Human Immunodeficiency Virus. The Journal of Alternative and Complementary Medicine.

Bowlby, J. (1973). Attachment and Loss: Vol. 2. Separation, Anxiety and Anger. Basic Books: New York.

Christian, L. M. (2012). Physiological reactivity to psychological stress in human pregnancy: Current knowledge and future directions. Elsevier.

Crusco, A., & Wetzel, C. (1984). The Midas Touch: the effects of interpersonal touch on restaurant tipping. Personality and Social Psychology Bulletin.

Culhane, J., Rauh, V., Farley-McCollum, K., Hogan, V., Agnew, K., & Wadhwa, P. D. (2001). Maternal stress is associated with bacterial vaginosis in human pregnancy. Elsevier.

Dada, R., Kumar, M., Jesudasan, R., Fernández, J., Gosálvez, J., & Agarwal, A. (2012). Epigenetics and its role in male infertility. Journal of Assisted Reproduction and Genetics.

Dalal K., Maran V., Pandey R., & Tripathi M, (2014) Determination of efficacy of reflexology in managing patients with diabetic neuropathy: a randomised controlled clinical trial. Evid Based Complement Alternat Med. 2014;2014:843036.

Daruna, J. H. (2012). Introduction to Psychoneuroimmunology. Academic Press.

DeAngelis, T., & Mwakalyelye, N. (1995). The power of touch helps vulnerable babies thrive. APA Monitor.

Demyttenaere, K., Nijs, P., Evers-Keibooms, G., & Koninckx, P. (1994). Personality Characteristics, psychoneuroendocrological stress and outcome depending upon the etiology of infertility. Gynecol Endocrinol.

DiPietro, J., Mendelson, T., Williams, E. L., & Costigan, K. (2011). Physiological Blunting during pregnancy extends to induced relaxation. Elsevier.

Ditzen, B., Neumman, L., Bodenmann, G., vonDawans, B., Turner, R., Ehlert, U., & Heinrichs, M. (2007). Effects of different kinds of couple interaction on cortisol and heart rate responses to stress in women. Psychoneuroimmunology.

Eaton, M., Mitchell-Bonair, I., & Friedmann, E. (1986) The effect of touch on nutritional intake of chronic organic brain syndrome patients. Journal of Gerontology.

Field, T., Hernandez-Reif, M., & Diego, M. (2005). Cortisol Decreases and Serotonin and Dopamine Increase Following Massage Therapy. University of Miami School of Medicine.

Fitzgerald, W. (1919) Zone Therapy, or Relieving Pain and Disease.

Fox, S. (2008). Relating to Clients. The Therapeutic Relationship For Complementary Therapists. London: JKP.

Fulkerson, M. (2014). The First Sense. A philosophical Study of Human Touch. MIT Press: Massachusetts.

Frankl, V, E., (1959) Man's Search for Meaning. Random House: Reading.

Gallace, A., & Spence, C. (2014). In Touch With the Future. The Sense of Touch from Cognitive Neuroscience to Virtual Reality. Oxford University Press: Oxford.

Galton, G. (2006). Touch Papers: Dialogues on touch in the psychoanalytic space. London: Karnac.

Gambles, M., Crooke, M., & Wilkinson, S. (2002). Evaluation of a hospice based reflexology service: a qualitative audit of patient perceptions. Eur. J. Oncol. Nurs.

Gazzola, V., Spezio, M., Etzel, J., Castelli, F., Adolphs, R., & Keysers, C. (2012). Primary somatosensory cortex discriminates affective significance in social touch. Proceedings of the National Academy of Sciences of the United States of America.

Genwei, W., & DongFang, H. (2006). Traditional Chinese Hand and Foot Massage. Beijing: Foreign Languages Press.

Geib, P. (1998). Touching in psychoanalytic practice. Wellington: The New Zealand Psychological Society.

Graham, H. (1999). Complementary Therapies in Context. London: JKP.

Grewen, K., Anderson, B., Girdler, S., & Light, K. (2003) Warm partner contact is related to lower cardiovascular reactivity. Behavioural Medicine.

Gueguen, N. (2004). Nonverbal encouragement of participation in a course: the effect of touching. Social Psychology of Education.

Han, B., Lee, H., Kim, T., Lim, J., & Shin, K. (2009). Tinnitus: Characteristics, Causes, Mechanisms, and Treatments. J Clin Neurol. Mar 2009; 5(1): 11–19.

Harlow, H. (1958). The Nature of Love. American Psychologist.

Hazel, C., & Perez, R. (2011). What Happens When You Touch The Body? The Psychology of Bodywork. Authorhouse.

Hertenstein, M., Holmes, R., McCullough, M., & Keltner, D. (2009). The communication of emotion via touch. Emotion.

Hertenstein, M., Keltner, D., App, B., Bulliet, B., & Jaskolka, A. (2006). Touch Communicates Distinct Emotions. Emotion.

Hold-Lunstad, J., Birmingham, W., & Light, K. (2008) Influence of a "Warm Touch" support enhancement intervention among married couples on ambulatory blood pressure, oxytocin, alpha amylase, and cortisol. Psychosomatic Medicine.

Honderich, T. (2005). The Oxford Companion to Philosophy. Oxford: Oxford University Press

Ingham, E. (1984) Revised Edition. Stories Feet Can Tell Thru Reflexology. Stories Feet Have Told Thru Reflexology. Ingham Publishing: Saint Petersburg.

Jang, S. H., & Kim, K. H. (2009). Effects of Self-Foot Reflexology on Stress, Fatigue and Blood Circulation in Premenopausal Middle-Aged Women. Korean Acad Nurs.

Ji, H., & Khurana Hershey, G., (2012) Genetic and epigenetic influence on the response to environmental particulate matter. American Academy of Allergy, Asthma & Immunology.

Jourard, S. (1966). An exploratory study of Body-Accessibility. British Journal of Social and Clinical Psychology.

Kaptchuk T, J. (2000), The Web That Has No Weaver. Chicago: Contemporary Books.

Keltner, D., (2007). http://greatergood.berkeley.edu/article/item/human_nature_redux_redux.

Kessler, R. C., Soukup, J., & Davis, R. B. (2001). The use of complementary and alternative therapies to treat anxiety and depression in the United States. American Journal of Psychiatry.

Kleinke, C. (1977). Compliance to requests made by gazing and touching experiments in field settings. Journal of Experimental Social Psychology.

Kress, I., Minati, L., Ferraro, S., & Critchley, H., (2012). Direct skin to skin vs indirect touch modulates neural responses to stroking vs tapping. Neurone port, 22, 646-651.

Lake, A. E. (2006), Medication Overuse Headache: Biobehavioural Issues and Solutions. Headache: The Journal of Head and Face Pain.

LeBon, T., (2001). Wise Therapy. London; Sage

Light, K., Grewen, K., & Amico, J. (2005) More Frequent Partner Hugs and Higher Oxytocin Levels are Linked to Lower Blood Pressure and Heart Rate in Premenopausal Women. Biological Psychology.

Lipton, B, H., (2008) Revised Edition. The Biology of Belief: Unleashing the Power or Consciousness, Matter & Miracles. London: Hay House LTD.

Loewer, B., (2008). 30 Second Philosophies. The 50 most thought-provoking philosophies, each explained in half a minute. London: Icon Books

Longrigg, J. (1993). Greek Rational Medicine. Philosophy and medicine from Alcmaeon to the Alexandrians. Routledge: Oxfordshire.

Lorenzo, G., Gomez C. (2004). Psychopathologic relationship between interstitial cystitis and rheumatic, autoimmune and chronic inflammatory diseases. The Journal of Spanish Urology, 57, 25-34.

Mackereth, P., Booth, K., Hillier, V., & Caress, A. (2009). What do people talk about during reflexology? Analysis of worries and concerns expressed during sessions for patients with multiple sclerosis. *Complementary Therapy Clin*.

Maddock, R., (1999). The retrosplenial cortex and emotion: new insights from functional neuroimaging of the human brain. Trends Neuroscience.

Manheimer, E., Zhang, G., & Udoff, L. (2008). Effects of acupuncture on rates of pregnancy and live birth among women undergoing in vitro fertilisation: systemic review and meta-analysis.

March-Smith, R. (2005). Counselling Skills for Complementary Therapists. London: Open University Press.

Mate, G. (2003). When The Body Says No. The Hidden Cost of Stress. Toronto: Vintage Canada.

McCabe, B. (1979). Autoimmune sensorineural hearing loss. Annals of Otology, Rhinology and Laryngology, 88, 585-589.

McCullough J., Liddle, S., Sinclair, M., Close, C., & Hughes, C. (2014). The Physiological and Biochemical Outcomes Associated with a Reflexology Treatment: A Systematic Review. Evidence-Based Complementary and Alternative Medicine.

McVicar, A, Greenwood CR, Fewell F, D'Arcy V, Chandrasekharan S, & Alldridge LC. (2007). Evaluation of anxiety, salivary cortisol and melatonin secretion following reflexology treatment: a pilot study in healthy individuals. Complementary Therapies in Clinical Practice. VOL 13; Number 3, page(s) 137-145.

Mitchell, A., & Cormack, M. (1998). The Therapeutic Relationship in Complementary Healthcare. Edinburgh: Churchstone Livingstone.

McGlone, F., Vallbo, A., Olausson, H., Loken, L., & Wessberg, J. (2007). Discriminative touch and emotional touch. Canadian Journal of Experimental Psychology. 61 (3), 173-183.

McLoud, J. (1998). An Introduction to Counselling. Buckingham: Open University Press.

McLeod, J. (2001). Qualitative Research in Counselling and Psychotherapy. London: Sage.

McLeod, S.A. (2008). Reductionism and Holism. Retrieved from http://www.simplypsychology.org/reductionism-holism.html

Mitchell, A., & Cormack, M. (1998). The Therapeutic Relationship in Complementary Healthcare. Edinburgh: Churchstone Livingstone.

Mearns, D. & Cooper, M., (2005). Working at Relational Depth in Counselling and Psychotherapy. London: Sage.

Monroe, C. (2009) The Effect of Therapeutic Touch on Pain. Journal of Holistic Nursing.

Moriam, S., & Sobhami, N. (2013). Epigenetic effect of chronic stress on Dopamine signalling and depression. Genetics and Epigenetics. 2013:5 11-16.

Nakamaru, T., Miura, N., Fukushima, A, & Kawashima, R. (2008). Somatotopical relationships between cortical activity, reflex areas in reflexology: A functional magnetic resonance imaging study. Neuroscience Letters. Volume 448, Issue 1, 19 December 2008, Pages 6-9.

Naoki, et al. (2013). Activity in the primary somatosensory cortex induced by reflexological stimulation is unaffected by pseudo-information: a functional magnetic resonance imaging study. BMC Complementary and Alternative Medicine. 2013. 13:11.

Paslow, R., Morgan, A. J., Allan, N. B., Jorm, A. F., O'Donnell, C. P., & Purcell, R. (2007). Effectiveness of complementary and self-help treatments for anxiety in children and adolescents. Medical Journal of Australia.

Prior, J. C. (1997). Ovulatory Disturbances: They Do Matter. Canadian Journal of Diagnosis.

Quattrin, R., Zanini, A., Buchini, S., Turello, D., Annunziata, M. A., Vidotti, C., et al. (2006). Use of Reflexology foot massage to reduce anxiety in hospitalised cancer patients in chemotherapy treatment: methodology and treatment. Journal of Nursing Management.

Ranabir, S., & Reetu K., (2011). Stress and hormones. Indian J Endocrinol Metab. 2011 Jan-Mar; 15(1): 18–22.

Rauschecker J, Leaver M, Mühlau M. 'Tuning Out the Noise: Limbic-Auditory Interactions in Tinnitus', Neuron, 2010; 66 (6): 819-826.

Rogers, C. (1951). Client-Centred Therapy. London: Constable.

Rutter, P. (1989). Sex in the forbidden zone. New York: St. Martins Press.

Ryff, C. D., & Singer, B. (2008). Know thyself and become what you are: A eudaimonic approach to psychological well-being. Journal of Happiness Studies, 9(1), 13-39.

Samuel. C., & Ebenezer I. (2013) Exploratory study on the efficacy of reflexology for pain threshold and tolerance using an ice-pain experiment and sham TENS control. Complementary Therapies in Clinical Practice.

Salvatore, P., Gariboldi, S., Offidani, A., Coppola, F., Amore, M., & Maggini, C. (2001). Psychopathology, personality and marital relationship in patients undergoing in vitro fertilisation procedures. Fertil Steril.

Sapolsky, R. M. (2004). Why Zebras Don't Get Ulcers, 3rd Edition. New York: St. Martins Press.

Schachter, S. & Singer, J.E. (1962). Cognitive, Social and Physiological Determinants of Emotional State.

Seemungal, B., Gresty, M., & Bronstein, A. (2001). The endocrine system, vertigo and balance. Current Opinion in Neurology. Vol 14 - Issue 1 - pp 27-34.

Seth, A., (2014) 30-Second Brain. The 50 most mind-blowing theories in neuroscience explained in half a minute. London: Icon Books.

Sliz, D., Smith, D., Wiebking, C., Northoff, G., & Hayley, S. (2012) Neural correlates of a single-session massage treatment. Brain Imaging and Behaviour. Volume 6, Issue 1, pp 77-87.

Smith, W. L., Clance, P.R., Imes, S. (1998). Touch in Psychotherapy – Theory, Research and Practice. Guildford Press: New York.

Stankiewicz, A, M., Swiergiel, A, & Lisowski, P. (2013). Epigenetics of stress adaptations in the brain. Brain Research Bulletin. September 2013, Vol.98:76–92.

Stenzel, C. L., & Rupert, P. A. (2004). Psychologists' use of touch in individual psychotherapy. Psychotherapy: Theory, Research, Practice, Training.

Stephenson, N., Dalton, J., & Carlson., J. (2003). The effect of foot reflexology on pain in patents with metastatic cancer. Applied Nursing Research. Vol 16 Issue 4, 284-286.

Stormer, C. (2007). The Language of the Feet. Oxen: Hodder Education.

Thompson, E. (2007). Mind in Life. Cambridge, MA: Harvard Press.

Tiran, D., & Mackereth, P. A. (2011). Clinical Reflexology. A Guide to Integrative Practice 2nd Edition. London: Churchstone Livingstone.

Tune, D. (2001). Is Touch a Valid Therapeutic Intervention? Counselling and Psychotherapy Research, BACP.

Traue, C. H, Bretzke, J. L, Pfingsten, M, Hrabal, V. Chapter Four: Psychological Factors in Pain Management. IASP.

Uehara, T., Yamasaki, T., Okamoto, T., Koike, T., Shigeyuki Kan, S., Satoru Miyauchi, S., Kira, J., & Shozo Tobimatsu, S. (2013). Efficiency of a "Small-World" Brain Network Depends on Consciousness Level: A Resting-State fMRI Study. Cereb. Cortex (2014) 24 (6): 1529-1539.

Uphoff-Chmiielnik, A. (1999). An exploration into touch in search of a rationale for its use within and as an adjunct to psychotherapy, with an emphasis on a person-centred model; or Beware – Here There Be Tiggers! Unpublished MA Dissertation, City University London.

Urich, R. S., Simons, R. F., Losito, B. D., Fiorito, E., Miles, M. A., & Zelson, M. (1991). Stress recovery during exposure to natural and urban environments. Journal of Environmental Psychology.

Van de Merwe, J. (2007). Interstitial cystitis and systemic autoimmune diseases. Nature Clinical Practice Urology, 4, 484-91.

Van Dijk, K., & Drzezga, A. (2014). The Default Network of the Brain. PET and SPECT in Neurology. 169-181.

Wadhwa, P. D. (2005). Psychoneuroendocrine processes in human pregnancy influence fetal development and health. Elsevier.

Weiss, S.J., Wilson, P., Hertenstein, M.J. & Campos, R.G. (2000). The tactile context of a mother's caregiving: Implications for attachment of low birth weight infants. Infant Behaviour and Development.

Williams, S., Clarke, D., & Gibson, K. (2011). The Use of Touch in Psychotherapy, A Thematic Analysis. Germany: Lambert.

Willis, F., & Hamm, H (1980). The use of interpersonal touch in securing compliance. Journal of Nonverbal Behaviour.

Wilson, A, G., (2008) Genetic and epigenetic influence on the response to environmental particulate matter. Academic Rheumatology Group, School of Medicine and Biomedical Sciences, University of Sheffield.

Wilson, K., & Ryan, Virginia. (2005) Second Edition. Play Therapy. A Non Directive Approach For Children And Adolescents. Oxford: Elsevier.

Whitcher, S., & Fisher, J. (1979) Multidimensional reaction to therapeutic touch in a hospital setting. Journal of Personality and Social Psychology.

Wong, J., Ghiasuddin, A., Kimata, C., Patelesio, B., & Siu, A. (2013). The impact of healing touch on paediatric oncology patients. Integrative Cancer Therapy.

http://www.livescience.com/37703-epigenetics.html.

http://neurosciencenews.com/neurogenetics-chronic-stress-health-572.

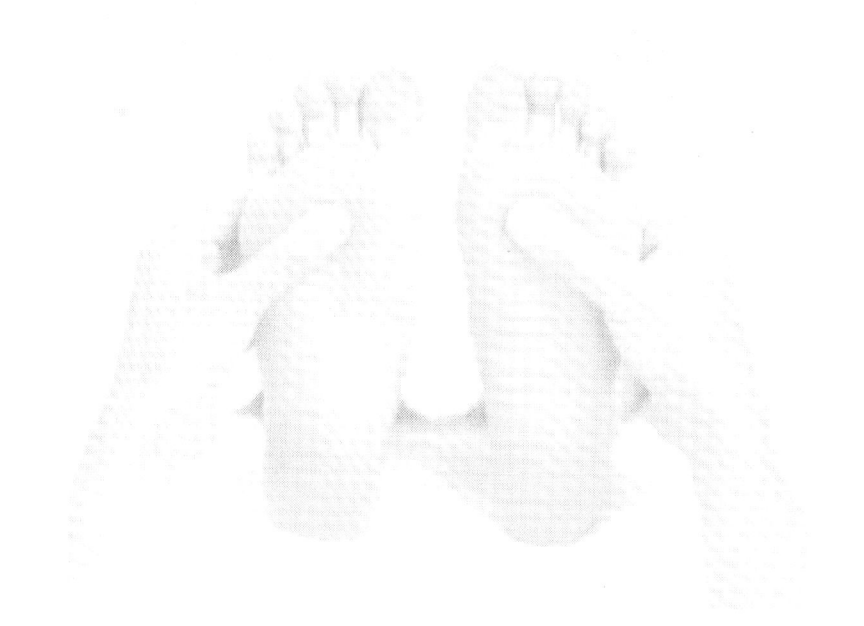

Relational Reflexology

Useful Links

Association of Reflexologists (AoR) (UK)	aor.org
Complementary and Natural Healthcare Council (CNHC) (UK)	cnhc.org.uk
Reflexology in Europe Network (RiEN)	reflexeurope.org
Judith Whatley	reflexscience.weebly.com
Greater Good Science Centre	greatergood.berkeley.edu
Migraine	migrainetrust.org
Interstitial Cystitis	cobfoundation.org
Sub-Fertility and IVF	hfea.gov.uk
Vertigo & Labyrinthitis	menieres.org.uk
Tinnitus	tinnitus.org.uk

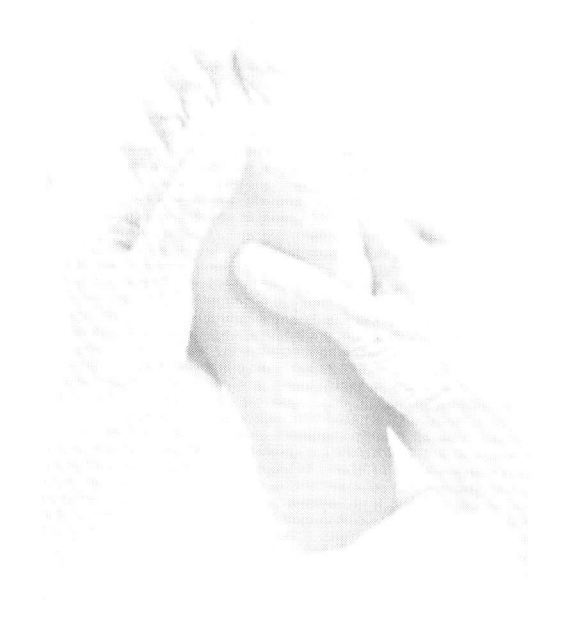

Relational Reflexology

Nichola Gregory MAR BA (Hons)

Nichola began her life in complementary therapies in 2005 when she initially trained as a professional reflexologist, quickly adding auricular acupuncture and hypnotherapy to her professional skills package. In her role as a complementary therapist Nichola has undertaken varied work, but is most experienced in the fields of chronic anxiety, migraine, and sub-fertility and supportive IVF.

In 2007, in response to her growing awareness of the complex and subtle connections between mind and body, Nichola embarked on an entry level counselling course, finally graduating as a professional counsellor in 2010.

As well as running her own private practice Nichola has provided counselling for a local G.P. practice, delivered one-to-one play therapy sessions for a national organisation working with emotionally vulnerable infant school children, and delivered reflexology and group acupuncture sessions within a national drug and alcohol service.

Nichola is a member of the Association of Reflexologists.

CPD FOR PROFESSIONAL REFLEXOLOGISTS

Nichola is the founder of **Relational Reflexology**; offering CPD training to qualified therapists focused upon enhancing practitioner self awareness and developing therapeutic relational skills. For further information please visit:

www.relationalreflexology.co.uk

Nichola blogs regularly about reflexology and her therapeutic work at:

www.relationalreflexology.wordpress.com

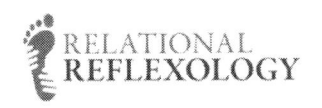

Made in the USA
Charleston, SC
05 September 2014